Caring for Dying Loved Ones

A HELPFUL GUIDE FOR FAMILIES AND FRIENDS

Joanna Lillian Brown

Caring for Dying Loved Ones™

Printed and published by
Levellers Press
Amherst and Florence, Massachusetts

www.levellerspress.com

ISBN 978-0-9819820-1-4

Author's website, including events, audio programs, additional
resources and blog: www.caringfordyinglovedones.com

Cover photo by *Patrick Zephyr* (www.patrickzephyr.com)
Author's photo by *Michael Zide* (www.michaelzide.com)

This book is lovingly dedicated to my former teacher

Beverly Hedison

Who instilled in me
A life-long love of learning

and to

George and Nancy Lower

Who embody what caregiving is all about.

Nancy became a quadriplegic in an accident in Africa while in the Peace Corps in 1999. Since that time, George and a dedicated band of friends and caregivers have cared for Nancy at home. Due to George's dedication and love, Nancy enjoys a life full of activities, such as bird club, singing in the choir, chairing the member care committee at her church, holding an opera subscription, and attending local baseball games. They travel widely, including visiting their four daughters and their partners/spouses and grandchildren.

TABLE OF CONTENTS

CHAPTER ONE

CHAPTER TWO

CHAPTER SIX

THE "DO IT NOW" LIST

CHAPTER SEVEN

HOSPICE CARE

CHAPTER THIRTEEN

To the Reader

This book is designed to be an easy-to-read book that introduces important concepts, issues, and options concerning caring for persons who are dying. It is not comprehensive, or it would be 600 pages, instead of 188 pages. If you need more information about topics or issues presented in this book, you will find a list of resources on pages 157–166, including books and web sites that can support you on your journey as a caregiver.

While I originally set out to write a book for caregivers, I have come to realize that this book can be useful for any person who wishes to ensure the highest quality of life for herself or himself in the last chapter of life. If you are reading this book for your own sake, I hope that you will find something useful, regardless of your current stage of life.

How to Use This Book

There is no right way to read this book. You may wish to read it straight through from front to back, or you might want to glance at the table of contents and turn to the chapter headings that call out to you. You might even want to open the book at random and see what is there on the page before you.

There are several forms within this book, to help you organize your thoughts. Feel free to copy these forms while they are blank, to put the forms into your "important notes" file or binder, or you can fill out the forms directly in the book to have them in one place.

Three Notes About Style

• In using the term "family" throughout this book, I do not want to imply that families have any particular configuration or that family members must be biologically related. Families can be biological or they can be "chosen," including persons who are friends, business associates, members of a religious or civic organization, or others who function as family. Throughout this book, family will refer to any individuals with a close connection to the dying person, whether or not they are related by blood or marriage.

•   I have chosen to intersperse the pronouns "he" and "she," or "his" and "her," throughout the text, to avoid using only the masculine pronoun "he" or the awkward constructs of "he/she" and "his/her." Please know that all of the situations described in this book can apply to someone of any gender.

•   Personal stories (my own or others) are set into *italics* to distinguish them from the "how to" tone of the surrounding text.

If You Are Already a Caregiver

If you are caring for a loved one whose health is declining or who has received a terminal diagnosis, this book will provide you with specific questions to consider and tangible steps to take at a time when your own mind may be too full of shock, grief, or panic to know how to be helpful to the person who is dying.

As a friend or relative of someone who is dying, you are in a unique position to be able to assist your loved one in thinking about a topic that most people fear—death—and in so doing, honor her wishes for how she wishes to live out her life.

Included in this book are two copies of a "My Wishes Survey," one for you, and one for your loved one. Taking the survey yourself will assist you in talking to your loved one about her wishes. If the ill or dying person is not capable of taking a survey, reflecting upon the person's life as you take the survey may help you to know what would enable him to have the highest quality of life in his last stage of living and dying.

If You Are Not Yet a Caregiver

If you are not yet helping someone who is dying, but you expect to become a caregiver to a loved one in the future, this book will help you to "think ahead," to go beyond the immediate stage in which you find yourself, in order to prepare yourself, emotionally and practically, for what is to come.

If Your Concern is Primarily About a Child

My own experiences form the foundation for this book. I am not a parent, and the caregiving situations in which I was involved did not include young children. Therefore, I have not attempted to address the issues concerning helping children in this book. If you need support in caring for a dying child or helping children within a family where someone is dying or has died, I encourage you to utilize the resources listed under "Children" on page 159 to find the information that you need.

A General Piece of Advice

The one piece of advice that I will give you, regardless of your circumstances, is to ask for support from others, whether from your spouse or partner, friends, relatives, members of a religious or civic organization to which you belong, volunteers or counselors at social service agencies, or a clergyperson, independent psychotherapist, psychologist, or social worker. Having someone to talk with is a great balm to the heart and spirit in times of stress and emotional pain.

CHAPTER TWO

Taking Your Own Temperature as a Caregiver

- Cool: Fine Now, but Looking Ahead to Future Responsibilities
- Warm: Facing Increasing Challenges of Caring for Someone
- Hot: Dealing with a Sudden Health Crisis
- Feverish Delirium: Being "In the Thick of It" and Feeling Overwhelmed

Taking your own temperature is a way of acknowledging what is happening for you at the present time and figuring out what you need to do next. The states described below: Cool, Warm, Hot, and Feverish Delirium, are not meant to imply that caregiving always escalates step by step to the point of feverish delirium, but these steps are offered as a way to validate the feelings that caregivers have at various times.

Cool: Fine Now, but Looking Ahead to Future Responsibilities

At this stage, you as a caregiver may have minimal ongoing responsibilities, but in your own mind you realize that there may come a time when your loved one will need your help to a greater extent.

Often the "cool" stage of caregiving involves gradual changes in your responsibilities, so gradual that you might not even acknowledge them as changes and probably don't feel them as burdensome. If the person whom you love doesn't live with you, such changes might include visiting or calling your loved one more frequently or making purchases for her via the internet or when you are already out shopping for yourself. If the loved one lives with you, you may instinctively begin to do more of the chores around the house or handle other tasks that had been hers.

Learning While You Can

If you are reading this book while your loved one is still relatively healthy and of reasonably sound mind, **you should know that one of the most unsettling changes that can happen when a health crisis does occur is that your loved one might lose his ability to speak or otherwise communicate with you, and this can be a permanent change.** I am bolding this statement because it deserves your full attention while he is still in reasonably good health.

Now is the time to learn from your loved one the skills that she knows and you do not know, for example, crocheting, lace making, playing cribbage, carving wood, playing a musical instrument, caring for trees or plants, or baking special recipes.

Look at and Label Photographs

If your loved one has collected family photographs in albums, but has not labeled them with captions, now is the time to review the photographs and caption as many as possible (either write on the back along an edge with a pencil or pen that won't show through, or tape a note to the back (do not use sticky notes, which will eventually fall off). If the photographs are still loose in shoe boxes or paper bags, take the time to review and sort the photos by approximate year or theme, putting groups of images into different envelopes and labeling the envelopes. Even if you do not have the time to put photographs into photo albums or scan them into a computer, if you are able to find out the names of at least some of the persons in the photograph, and the event depicted, you will have accomplished a most important task in saving your family history. *I say this with regret— many of our family photographs never were labeled before my parents were no longer able to help with this task, and the persons in the photographs will be anonymous forever.*

Record Their Stories via Tape Recording, Video Recording, or Taking Notes

Some persons have within them a treasure trove of stories about their own lives and their ancestors' lives. If you wish to preserve any of this history about your family and how life was lived long ago— stories of the "old country"; how they or their grandparents or great grandparents immigrated (were they part of a diaspora or were they forceably brought here during the slave trade?); stories of life on the farm, in the coal mines, in the shipyards, or in the factories and tenement houses; life in the days of horse drawn carriages and "ice boxes," before radio, television, telephones, and computers—now is the time to record their stories for posterity.

I am grateful that my sister thought to videotape my grandmother one day when she and I and a cousin were visiting with our grandmother in her kitchen. We told our grandmother that we had a camera on a tripod so we could take a few photographs. We did, indeed, pose for a few still photographs, but we also left the video camera on, and it recorded our completely unrehearsed conversations and instructions from our grandmother about how to make a favorite dessert. That videotape is now one of our family's prized possessions.

Please do not put off this activity of recording oral history and special stories, assuming that you can do it another time, for you cannot estimate how much time your loved one has on this earth, or for how much longer she will have a good enough memory to tell you her stories and identify people in photographs. Whether you capture these stories via voice recording, video recording, or by hiring someone else to interview your loved one, you will always be glad that you took the time to do this (you can search via the web to find professional memoir writers in your area).

Not Fully Living, but Not Yet Dying

Often, before someone begins to die, they enter a state that I describe as *not fully living, but not yet dying.* In this phase, which can last for months or years, the elderly or ill person loses the ability to do and enjoy many of the things that he ordinarily would want to do. Whereas in the past he had enjoyed cooking and eating with great gusto, he might begin to eat only frozen or canned food, or may only eat snack foods. Whereas she might have enjoyed regular physical activities or doing crafts, she may become completely sedentary.

Loss of Prior Activities and Interests

Persons in this not fully living, not yet dying phase of life may stop doing the intellectual, cultural, and creative activities that they once enjoyed, whether going to the theater and concerts, reading books or newspapers, doing crafts or handiwork, or participating in civic and community events. This lack of interest can be due to gradual loss of hearing or sight, the inability to drive, increasing dementia or physical illness, the death or illness of a spouse, or the unraveling of their network of friends, as the friends move away, are no longer able to communicate, become ill, or die.

Talking to your loved one about her former activities and interests may provide information that allows you to find a solution to her problem—a neighbor or who can take her to a concert or civic meeting, an elder van to bring him to the local senior center for specific activities, or rotating responsibilities among family members and friends to make sure that he has opportunities to continue the activities that are of interest to him.

New Interests or Interests Intensifying

Although in this stage the person's world is gradually becoming smaller, new interests may emerge or old interests can intensify. *One friend's mother had loved being outdoors and going on long walks to watch the birds. Although she could no longer go on walks outside, in her last stage of life she watched birds visiting her bird feeder with greater intensity, and this became the focal point of her daily routine.*

Working with Diminished Abilities in New Ways

My mother had always enjoyed doing the crossword puzzle in the daily newspaper and in crossword puzzle books. In her 80s, crossword puzzles gained increased importance, to the point that in the last few years of her life, most of her waking hours were spent doing crossword puzzles in puzzle magazines.

Even though her ability to solve new puzzle clues began to fail, we realized that her long-term memory could recall words used in previous crossword puzzles. She could still remember answers to obscure clues such as "three letter word for cleric's robe"—"alb," she said, proudly. "I know that!"

Seeing that she could still solve the puzzles in puzzle books that she had done in the past, my sibling ordered many copies of one old puzzle book. This enabled her to draw on her long-term memory to successfully solve the puzzles, yet because of her loss of short-term memory, she never realized that she was doing the same puzzle book over and over again. This is one example of how careful observation can allow you to capitalize on your loved one's strengths and compensate for the loss of abilities, in order to find activities that your loved one can still enjoy.

Invest Your Time in Thinking About and Preparing for the Future

The diminishment of your loved one's interests and intellectual and physical capacities should be a signal to you that she will need additional help in the future. This is the stage where you, as a loved one and potential caregiver, would be well-served to *invest* some of your time (rather than *spending* your time) in learning concepts, skills, and tasks that will have considerable pay-back in the months and years ahead:

• Read the "Do It Now" chapter that begins on page 63. This is a wonderful time to ask him about the existence of a will and power of attorney documents, so you can learn if these documents exist and what information is contained in them. If your loved one does not wish to talk about funeral plans, do not force the issue. You may be able to find out some of his preferences for what might be in a memorial service by asking questions of a more general nature, such as "Who is your favorite musician or singer, Dad?" or, "What are some of the best books that you have read?"

• Be sure to go along with your loved one to all doctors' appointments, or have another trusted person do so. When your loved one is at this stage, you cannot trust that she can understand and remember information that she may receive in a medical appointment, and many doctors do not take the time to check to see if a patient understands what they say. *A friend of mine was shocked to see that her mother seemed to ignore a doctor's warning about the importance of taking a certain medication. She turned to her mother and said, "Mom, did you hear what the doctor said? He said that if you don't take your medicine and your heart doesn't become regulated within the next few days, you will die." At that moment, her mother put her hand in the air and said, "I am not ready to die!" Her mother began taking the medication and lived another nine months.*

• Have some informal conversations with your loved one concerning what quality of life means to him or her, utilizing some or all of the questions in the "My Wishes" survey on pages 44–53.

• Get a File of Life form and its small plastic pouch in which to keep it, to attach to the front of your refrigerator for each person living in the house. This form and pouch contain emergency contact information for next of kin and the medical health agent, as well as information about existing medical conditions, allergies, current medications and dosages. Be sure to make copies of the File of Life form for the health care agent, the alternate agent, and an additional person, such as someone living closest to the ill person. In this way, this important information can always be accessed in an emergency situation. File of Life forms are usually distributed by local Councils on Aging, Senior Centers, Fire Departments, or Police Departments.

• This is also a good time to ask about the existence of health care proxy and living will documents, so that you can learn if they already exist, and where they are kept. (See the "Do It Now" list of documents on page 63). It is a good idea, for everyone, not only aging or dying people, to review these documents every five years to make sure that persons listed as the medical health care agent and alternate are not deceased or unable to serve.

I was lucky enough to raise these topics with my parents before either had declined to a great degree. I discovered that my parents' will had named a long-deceased lawyer as their power of attorney and executor of their estate, and that no alternate power of attorney or executor had been named. Our conversations enabled me to suggest that my parents review and update all of their legal documents and their health care proxy and living will forms, which they did. Having these actions taken care of before either of them declined in health to the point of not being able to do so was a great relief to me.

• Read the next chapter to think about what you want your role as a caregiver to be. Talk to your spouse, partner, significant other, siblings, in-laws, children, friends or anyone else whom you consider to be close to your loved one to learn their thoughts about what they would want their roles as caregivers to be.

• Investigate some of the resources listed on pages 157–166 and think about options for end of life care, before a crisis forces you to do so on short notice. Whatever you do now in terms of educating yourself about some general issues—medical, psychological and spiritual—with dying persons, as well as learning specific information about whatever medical conditions your loved one has, will pay dividends later on, when you may not have the time to learn about the issues facing you.

Warm: Facing Increasing Challenges of Caring for Someone

This stage is what I call the long slippery slope of caregiving. As time goes by, you may find yourself re-arranging your own schedule to make your visits to an ill or aging parent or friend more frequent and intentional and less impromptu. The quality of your time spent with this person may also change, as visits focus less on discussing shared topics of interest and more on his health problems, your concerns about him, or the tasks that need to be done.

Shifting Roles and Responsibilities

If the person who is ailing is a spouse, partner, or other person who is living with you, you may feel the relationship shift from being equals to experiencing that more of the responsibilities that she used to have are now being shifted to your shoulders, without first discussing and agreeing upon this. You may begin to do more cooking, laundry, housecleaning, lawn mowing, child care, or bill paying than you had in the past, and these additional tasks may be begin to feel burdensome to you.

If the ill person fails to acknowledge the increased responsibilities you are shouldering, you may begin to feel unappreciated or resentful. Alternately, the ill person who is aware that responsibilities are being taken from him may begin to feel a loss of control or status and resent you for doing tasks "that are his to do."

If you feel that you are in the "Warm" phase, at any time the situation could change from stable to unstable. **As I have already listed in the "Cool" phase on page 6, one of the most unsettling changes that can happen as your loved one declines in health is that she can lose her ability to reason, speak, or otherwise communicate with you, and this can be a permanent change.**

Before your loved one loses the ability to communicate with you, or you face a crisis that will turn everything upside down, taking a few steps to prepare for what is to come can truly serve you. The steps you will want to consider taking in this phase (in addition to the ones listed in the "Cool Phase" on pages 5–11), are:

• Read the chapter entitled the "Do it Now List" and begin conversations with your loved one about these important documents. Ask your loved one if his will, health care proxy, and power of attorney documents exist, and review and update those documents (or create ones if they do not already exist). This task should be on the top of your personal "to do" list.

• Have conversations with your loved one concerning what quality of life means to him or her, utilizing some or all of the questions in the "My Wishes" survey. (See pages 33–53)

• If you have not already done so, get a File of Life form and its small plastic pouch in which to keep it, to attach to the front of your refrigerator for each person living in the house. This form and pouch contain the person's full name and address, emergency contact information for next of kin and the medical health agent, as well as information about the person's primary care physician, existing medical conditions, allergies, current medications and dosages, and which physician prescribed which medication. If you do not have a File of Life form, you can list the above information, as well as the person's date of birth, Medical Insurance company and policy number, Medicare or Medicaid ID number, any other special notes or conditions, and the person's religion (if appropriate). Be sure to make copies of the File of Life form for the health care agent, the alternate agent, and an additional person, such as someone living closest to the ill person. In this way, this important information can always be accessed in an emergency situation. File of Life forms are usually distributed by local Councils on Aging, Senior Centers, Fire Departments, or Police Departments.

• Explore options for in-home service providers to allow you to get a sense of the availability of services, who the various vendors are, and the range of services and costs associated with them. Many towns and cities have a Council on Aging or an elder care services agency that can either provide in-home services or make referrals to them.

- Begin to familiarize yourself with the hospices in your area. You can check your phone book or internet listings for local visiting nurses associations (VNA) that also do hospice care, or you can check for listings of hospices in the White or Yellow Pages (which may be listed in the white pages under the city name (for example, Springfield VNA and Hospice), an organization name (for example, Hospice Life Care of (county or city), or as a listing under the local hospital as a department or service). Sometimes there will be more than one hospice that will serve a given area. Now is the time to see what educational programs each hospice offers and attend a lecture or presentation. This will not only increase your understanding about hospice services, but will allow you to meet the staff of the hospice and decide which agency might better meet your needs down the road.

- Chose a specific file folder or other location for collecting information that you find in your research, and put everything you find into it. I have found that a plastic or paper accordion file with many different sections is most useful, so that you can label the different sections for different types of documents or notes. I chose a brightly colored file folder, to make it easier to find even when it is amidst other documents or folders. Accordion files and other types of folders are available at stationery and office supply stores, in the stationery sections of supermarkets, or through online vendors.

- Purchase an 8.5 by 11 (or 6 by 9) inch spiral bound notebook in which family members can enter notes, observations, and questions while visiting. This can be kept in a specific drawer that is not in general use by your loved one or other visitors, to maintain the privacy of your remarks. You will really come to appreciate this history of how and when things began to change as your loved one progresses through the last chapter of his life.

- As you talk with several organizations concerning housekeeping services, home health aides, and visiting nurse services, write notes on a different page for each service provider. Be sure to record the date and time of your conversation, the name of the person with whom you spoke, and the important information that they gave you, so that you can quickly reference the information in the future and can ask to speak to the same person. (**See the template contact form on pages 16 –17, and make as many copies of it as you need for**

your use.) Be sure to note the minimum hours the service provider will work (for example, two hours at a time) and whether travel time is included in the cost or is billed as an additional cost. Most agencies offer different hourly rates for different levels of service provided. It is not necessary to pay for a nurse when a housekeeper or certified nursing assistant (CNA) is all that is needed. Moreover, a licensed practical nurse (LPN) might be qualified to administer the treatment that your loved one needs. If so, the cost per visit or per hour will probably be less expensive than if you hire a registered nurse (RN).

Having initial conversations with several different agencies or service providers will also give you needed information about how responsive the agency is. I have long believed that the first interactions with any service provider, whether doctor, psychotherapist, dentist, home-care agency, or funeral home, tell you a great deal about them. If the person answering the phone is calm, collected, and helpful, this is a good indication. If the person is harried, short-tempered, and places you on hold for a long period of time, this does not bode well for the quality of service you will receive later on. I urge you to take notes about any unsatisfactory interactions, rather than making excuses for any rude behavior or poor service. Finding reliable, courteous, helpful providers with a commitment to quality care takes time and effort, but that effort will be time well spent if you can feel confident that the service will be reliable and the administrative staff will be responsive.

• If your loved one is still cogent and active, but mildly forgetful, make sure that there is a card with his or her name and address, telephone number and emergency contact name and phone number inside the pocket of his coats, as well as in his wallet. In case the coat is left at the senior center, or in case he has an accident, this information will be readily available.

• Investigate if there is a "Village to Village" self-help membership organization in your area, or start one if there isn't. (Go to the web site www.vtvnetwork.org.) The first nonprofit neighborhood "village" organization started in 2001 in Beacon Hill in Boston, but there are more than 50 in existence as of 2010, with the number growing each year. These mutual-aid societies, funded with membership dues, offer free handyman services, rides to the food market, and companionship to persons 50 or older who wish to stay in their homes but are no longer self-sufficient. Many of these villages are located in expensive areas of cities or suburbs, but the concept could have much wider applicability, if it were to be adopted by area Councils on Aging and hospices. Whether this self-help movement continues to grow remains to be seen, but this is one of the most promising developments in end of life care that I have heard about in the last few years.

• If you begin to feel confused, anxious, or fearful about the responsibilities that you are encountering, talking with trusted friends or hospice volunteers may offer sufficient advice and support. If talking to friends does not alleviate these symptoms, seek the counsel of a professional psychotherapist or counselor in order to better understand your feelings and thoughts about these shifting roles and responsibilities. When deciding on which professional to see, ask if they have experience in assisting clients with caregiving and end of life issues. If the dying person is your spouse, consulting with a couples counselor will give you a better idea of whether counseling could be helpful to both of you as a couple, or just you as an individual. Regardless of what your relationship is to the dying person, counseling can help you if fear, anxiety, worry, depression, anger, or any strong emotions are beginning to take hold of you in a way that is not productive for you.

Provider Contact Form:

(You may wish to copy this form before filling it out)

Agency/Organization: _____

Website: _____

Address: _____

City _____

State _____   Zip _____

PhoneNumber(s):_____

Date of contact:_____ Time of contact:_____

Person whom I contacted:

_____

Type of services offered:

_____

_____

_____

_____

_____

_____

_____

Costs of services, minimum hours, other items of note:

_____

_____

_____

_____

_____

Next steps to take:

_____

_____

_____

_____

Additional notes:

Date/Time   Contact Person   Subject

_____

_____

_____

_____

_____

Hot: Dealing with a Sudden Health Crisis

Sometimes, bad things happen unexpectedly. Dad, who was healthy only two weeks ago, falls and breaks his hip. Or your spouse or partner has a sudden stroke leading to incapacitation. This is a three-alarm emergency that requires many decisions to be made at once, or in a very short time frame, at best. Usually, the first step after a crisis is that the person is admitted to the hospital for evaluation and stabilizing treatment. Since hospitals are now under such pressure from insurers to release patients at the earliest possible moment, the window of time in which to plan your next steps can be extremely short, from as little as a few hours to as long as two or three days.

The first thing that you want to train yourself to do is to "document, document, document." Choose a notebook where you can begin to record all incidents, events, and conversations that you have with others, noting the date, time, content and persons involved. If you don't do this, the blur of activity will swirl around you and you will quickly forget with whom you have spoken, and about what, and who promised to do which thing that needs to be done.

Call an Emergency Family Meeting

Now is the time to convene a family meeting, preferably face-to-face. *As a friend of mine said, "Don't accept 'I'm too busy' as an answer from other family members. It's our mother and these are our decisions. I don't want to hear 'I'm too busy,' no matter how far away you are."* If necessary, a conference call or Skype (phone-video call) can take the place of an initial meeting, but having everyone in the same room to talk about what will happen next is far superior to having only voice or email communication. You will want to be able to look everyone in the eye and see the dynamics happening in the room as you discuss these important issues.

Request and Review Your Loved One's Medical Records

Medical mistakes happen all of the time. Grab that File of Life from the refrigerator door and bring the written list of your loved one's medications to the emergency room. *A friend of mine told me two hair raising stories that had happened to his father. Once, his father had a fall and was taken to the emergency room. He verbally told the medical personnel that his father was on a certain prescription medicine (beginning with the letter "A") twice a day. The medical intake person incorrectly heard what he had said and wrote down a similar sounding, but completely different, medication. The next day that they visited him in the hospital, the father was almost comatose, requiring immediate treatment to offset the response to the wrong drug.*

That is not where the errors ended. The doctors recommended inserting a drug-treated stent into one of his arteries. Luckily, the family member knew that his father was allergic to aspirin, and that the drug coating the stent was related to aspirin. "Not to worry," the doctors said. They could "desensitize" the father to aspirin over the course of a day or two. However, they never notified the family that this treatment would cause a diabetic-like condition for those days of treatment. Not knowing this, the family was happy to bring an ice cream sundae, at the father's request, which he promptly ate. This put him into an emergency condition requiring immediate insulin treatment, and his condition did not stabilize for many days thereafter.

All people receiving medical treatment (and their appointed health care agents) need to be fully informed about the effects of their medications, possible allergic responses, and any other information that could have a bearing on further treatment, and the persons who care about them need to act as advocates to ensure that medical mistakes do not happen.

NOTE: the Health Insurance Portability and Accountability Act of 1996 (known as HIPAA) was passed to protect the privacy of individually identifiable health care information. When your loved one enters the hospital or a nursing home, you will be required to fill out a HIPAA form to indicate who should have access to your loved one's medical records. See page 162 in the resource section for the US Department of Health and Human Services website where you can learn about HIPAA rules and print out a copy of the HIPAA "Authorization for Disclosure of Protected Health Information" form.

Whether your loved one is being cared for in the hospital, a rehabilitation facility, nursing home or at home, having a spiral bound notebook that is kept in a bureau drawer or night table stand, where family members can make notes on conversations with medical personnel, medications added or changed, and significant observations about the loved one's mental and physical capabilities, will be an invaluable resource, as family members come and go on different shifts of caregiving.

If you hire in private duty nurses, certified nursing assistants, or others, have a separate (smaller, and different color) notebook where you ask hired staff to print their name, start and end times, and observations, on each shift they work, and in which family members can write instructions or questions for the paid caregivers.

Clear the Deck of Other Responsibilities

Whatever you can do to eliminate other responsibilities in your life, such as arranging for child care, taking time off from work, arranging for pet sitting or kenneling your dog or cat, I hope that you will do that now. Your priorities at this point are as follows:

• Communicate immediately with your loved one's current health care providers, to inform them about the health crisis taking place and to make sure that lists of medications and dosages, as well as allergies, are faxed or sent to the hospital, so that doctors, specialists, and other providers who may be caring for your loved one at the present time will avoid medication errors and dangerous drug interactions or complications.

• Communicate immediately with other close relatives or friends, to inform them about the situation at hand and to arrange for a joint meeting, in person or via phone or internet, to discuss future options. Create a list of their names, home/work/cell/pager phone numbers, email addresses, and mailing addresses, and then email or send that list to everyone else on the list. It can be extremely helpful to set up a group email list or a Facebook page (www.facebook.com) so that you can update many persons at once. You might also consider launching a web page at www.caringbridge.org. This nonprofit organization makes web pages available to families dealing with chronic or acute medical illness. If you are not familiar with setting up a group email list or Facebook or Caringbridge web page, ask relatives or friends, or someone at the nearest Senior Center or Council on Aging, if they can assist you.

- Check to see if Medical Proxy and Power of Attorney documents exist, and review them with the person who is ill, if it is possible to do so. If the ill person is not able to communicate, and the documents are out of date or missing altogether, consult with a lawyer to find out if it is possible via a court hearing to have a judge appoint you or someone else, on a temporary basis, to serve as Attorney in Fact and/or Medical Proxy.

- Decide who from the family will be the primary contact person with the medical staff, and notify the medical staff of this decision. Oftentimes it is best to have the person who is designated as the medical proxy be the primary contact person, so that important decisions can be made quickly. Designating one person as the primary contact person is important because it is difficult for health care staff to have many different family members calling to ask questions, and it is confusing for the medical staff to not know whom to call when questions arise or important information needs to be given to the family.

- Decide who in the cluster of family or friend caregivers will take on the following responsibilities, and **write down the name and the responsibility to which they have agreed** (don't rely on your memory or someone else's) and **then email or send them to everyone who should know who is doing what.**

  - Contacting other family members and friends
  - Contacting the person's employer or business associates, if appropriate
  - Alerting the person's clergyperson or other spiritual advisor
  - Alerting the person's landlord or close neighbors about her absence and giving them your contact information. This is so someone can keep an eye on the property for you and also so that they do not mistakenly call the police if they do not see your relative do her predictable routines, such as raising or lowering the shades, going out to get her newspaper, or checking her mailbox
  - Taking care of animals
  - Canceling "Meals on Wheels" or any other recurring services that are currently in place and are not needed
  - Paying bills such as mortgage, rent, utilities
  - Watering plants

- Arranging with the post office for mail to be held or forwarded to another address
- Temporarily suspending, or canceling, delivery of a daily newspaper
- Picking up and returning voice messages on the person's phone or answering machine
- Changing an outgoing answering message or having all calls forwarded from the person's phone to another number
- Temporarily adjusting the thermostat and/or hot water heater to reduce utility costs

- If there is no one else living at the person's home or apartment, discuss what each person will do to secure the property, such as:
  - Checking to make sure all windows and doors are locked
  - Closing, or partially closing, some blinds or curtains
  - Running the garbage disposal, removing trash from all rooms, and making sure that toilets are flushed
  - Checking to make sure that the stove is not on and any appliances such as automatic coffee percolators are turned off
  - Turning off alarm clock or radio-alarm clock alarm settings, especially if the person lives in an apartment building where such settings could disturb others if left unattended
  - Removing any perishable food from counters and the refrigerator (be sure to check inside the microwave oven and regular oven, too)
  - Installing timers on one or more lights, and also perhaps on a radio or television

Feverish Delirium: Being "In the Thick of It" and Feeling Overwhelmed

Perhaps you have come to this book during the stage when you feel as if everything, or nearly everything, is in flux. It is easy to feel overwhelmed at this point, especially if you are the primary care provider for the person who is ill or dying.

I urge you to read the steps outlined in the "Cool" and "Warm" sections that are immediately before this one, in order to see what practical steps could help you. In addition, you will need to focus on specific ways to maintain your own health and wellbeing as you encounter highly stressful situations on an ongoing basis.

Find Ways to Get More Support and Bring Balance to Your Life

The most important goal for you, if you are feeling overwhelmed, is to find ways to get more support and bring more balance to your life, so that you survive this difficult time. It may seem obvious to others, but not to you, that if you "crash and burn" in your attempt to do more than you are capable of doing, you may become vulnerable to illness or have an accident. This will not only take its toll on you but will deprive your loved one of your presence and your caregiving. Be sure to set aside some time each week that is dedicated to your own rest and renewal, even if you think that you do not need to do so.

An example from my own family will illustrate this point. When my grandmother was dying in 1991, my mother, who lived upstairs from my grandmother, was her daily helper. As a person who also was a caregiver for my grandmother, I could see that my mother was looking more and more exhausted, yet she denied needing any help. One day, when my mother was hanging out the laundry on the back porch, something that she had done many times before, she fainted, falling face first onto the sidewalk about four feet below her. Miraculously, she only suffered bad bruises and sprains, but her injuries were disabling enough that we decided to place my grandmother in a nearby nursing home for several days of respite care so that my mother could rest and heal herself.

My grandmother's experience in the nursing home was not a positive one, and we brought her back to her home as soon as we were able to arrange for increased support from family members and private duty certified nursing assistants so that my mother would not overextend herself again.

Some of the actions that will help you to "give care to the caregiver" at this stage are:

•   Be intentional about getting sufficient rest.

•   Eat healthy foods on a regular schedule. Skipping meals because you are too busy is not a strategy that will maintain your energy.

•   Build into your schedule some appointments to do things you love to do, either alone or with people whom you enjoy. Whether you love to go the movies, see live theater, play a game of tennis, watch a ball game, take a walk, read books, or have lunch at a particular restaurant, intentionally schedule times away from caregiving for yourself or with your spouse, partner, or friends. Taking your mind off of your responsibilities and off of your worries will help to recharge your batteries.

• Discuss with your family members having them sign up for specific shifts of care, or having them pay for the care, if they do not want to, or cannot, give the care themselves. You should plan to have one day off from caregiving per week, when you do not need to give the direct care or worry about who is giving the care.

• Set aside some time for spiritual and physical replenishment. Taking even ten or fifteen minutes to read an inspirational book, pray or meditate, do yoga, exercise, or walk in an area that you love will restore your energy and calm your mind.

• If you are exhausted, consider your options for enlisting respite care. If the dying person is living with you, you may want to consider having him be temporarily admitted to a facility for short-term care, or you can bring in private duty help (or family volunteers) and take a vacation. You will probably restore yourself more deeply if you leave the immediate area, rather than staying in the same house, or even nearby.

Your mind may play tricks on you and tell you that you do not need to do anything that is "fun," during such a serious time. Ignore such a voice if you hear it! The challenges before you will be even greater, and it is in your best interest, as well as the best interest of your loved one, if you occasionally step off of the treadmill of your life as a caregiver and do something with an entirely different focus and rhythm.

CHAPTER THREE

What Do I Want My Role To Be As a Caregiver?

- Factors to Consider
- Peer Support and Counseling
- Places on the Caregiving Spectrum
- Being the Primary Caregiver
- Responsibilities and Accountabilities
- Helping from Afar
- Appreciating and Supporting the Primary Caregiver

Factors to Consider

If you are facing the prospect of helping someone who is dying, the most important question for you to consider is: What do I want my role to be as a caregiver?

There are two other factors that may help you to come to some clarity about your answer: your own health and your own attitudes about death and dying.

Your Own Health

If your own health is not strong, I suggest that you have a physical examination to check your general health and any medical conditions that are specific to you, and to discuss your potential caregiving role with your own health practitioner. Being informed about your own health status, and taking the steps to correct any imbalances that are found, will allow you to be realistic about your own caregiving capacities and prevent a health care crisis of your own.

Your Own Attitudes about Death and Dying

Death is one of the subjects that is "taboo" in our culture. If you are anxious or fearful about helping a dying person, you can educate yourself about aspects of death and dying by reading books and looking at websites listed in the reference section on page 157–166. It is also helpful to talk with volunteers or staff members at a hospice who have been through what you are going through. These volunteers and staff members can share their experience with you and answer questions that you may have, and thus lessen your fear of the unknown.

I found that being with my grandmother at her death was a very spiritual experience that removed my fear of dying. I now share my experiences of being with loved ones at the time of their deaths with friends and colleagues who are approaching a caregiving role, so that they can be encouraged to offer support and love to their family members and friends. This is a case where, in the words of Franklin Delano Roosevelt, "The only thing we have to fear is fear itself."

Peer Support and Counseling

Whether your relationship with your loved one is positive or laced with difficulties, you may experience strong emotions surfacing at this time. If so, I encourage you to consider sharing your feelings with a trusted friend or availing yourself of professional counseling.

Talking with a trusted friend offers several advantages. First, he or she will offer support at no cost, and you can arrange to speak when it is convenient for both of you, often on short notice. Second, the person already knows you and may also know your family members or others close to the dying person. Your friend may simply provide a listening ear, or she may have advice to share with you, based on her own experiences.

If you do reach out to a friend for support, keep in mind that he may or may not be available at the time that you need help, or he may not be ready or able to talk with you about matters pertaining to death and dying. If he declines your invitation to talk to you, do not take the rejection personally. Many people have not had the experience of being with someone as they have died, and your friend may not feel prepared to be the one you turn to for advice and support.

If a close friend is not willing or able to be your confidante, or if simply having access to a good listener is not sufficient, I encourage you to seek an individual counselor or clergyperson to help you deal with your feelings. Of course, if you experience strong emotions that interfere with your daily living, such as confusion, depression, anger, or anxiety, then this is not a situation in which you should rely on support from a friend. This is the time to seek professional guidance from a licensed counselor, social worker, psychotherapist, psychologist, psychiatrist, or clergyperson.

Seeing a professional counselor or clergyperson will guarantee you confidentiality, and knowing that your thoughts will remain private can lessen the anxiety of opening up yourself to difficult emotions and memories.

There are many counselors who specialize in various types of short-term counseling. It is not necessary to sign on to a lengthy process of traditional, "on the couch" Freudian analysis to gain insights to support your decision making and take the steps you need as a caregiver.

If you work for a company or organization that offers an Employee Assistance Plan (EAP), you could qualify for a certain number of free, confidential counseling sessions. Check with your Human Resources Office about such a benefit and a referral to a list of qualifying counselors.

If you do not have an EAP at your workplace, you can find a list of counselors in the Yellow Pages under "Counseling-Personal and Family," or you can call your local United Way agency to ask if they sponsor a social services locator number (usually "211") that can be dialed from any phone, toll-free in your area for a confidential referral to counselors of all types.

Counselors have different titles, depending on their type of training: psychiatrists (those with a medical degree and specialization in psychology); psychologists (those with a doctoral degree in psychology), psychotherapists (also referred to as therapists, who generally have a master's degree in psychology or clinical counseling), licensed clinical social workers (those with a masters degree in social work), or marriage and family counselors (who will have a master's degree or higher in psychology or clinical counseling). Be sure to ask how much experience the counselor has dealing with the issues you wish to discuss (such as helping people who dying). This is no time to be the counselor's first client who needs support around end of life issues!

If you have never been to a counselor before, you should know that it is perfectly all right to talk to several counselors, on the phone or in person, before making up your mind which one would be right for you. Service providers should be willing to tell you (by phone or in person, or through printed information or a web site) about their training, their areas of specialty, the type of counseling that they do with clients, how much they charge per session, and whether their services are covered by your insurance plan, before you decide to see them on a paying basis.

Places on the Caregiving Spectrum

There are many places in the spectrum of caregiving, from being the primary caregiver (and the coordinator of other caregivers), to being one of several frequent caregivers, to being an occasional caregiver, to handling responsibilities other than direct care (such as bill paying), to being a frequent visitor, to visiting occasionally and communicating with the dying person and their loved ones via phone, email, website, or correspondence.

Being the Primary Caregiver

In my experiences helping loved ones in the final stages of their lives, I have found that there is usually one person who either consciously takes on the role of being the primary caregiver, or who ends up being the primary caregiver (because no one else is available or is willing to do it). Being a primary caregiver means that you are the person who will help the dying person most frequently, perhaps daily, perhaps even on a live-in basis, and you may also be the one who will coordinate other care workers.

If you choose to take on the role of being the primary caregiver, you will shoulder much of the burden of caregiving, perhaps leaving you with little time for your own interests or for your family life. You will also reap the benefits of being present during remarkable moments—moments of love, vulnerability, and laughter— that other members of the family will miss, and you will probably develop a special level of closeness with the dying person.

Being a primary caregiver is both a burden and a blessing, but I have yet to meet someone who served in that role who regretted doing so. The guidance in this chapter is meant to ease your journey and encourage you to take good care of yourself, even in the most challenging times.

Responsibilities and Accountabilities

In addition to giving direct care to the dying person, there are many roles to take if you do not wish to do direct physical care but wish to take on some responsibilities.

These other non-caregiving roles include:

- Coordinating caregivers
- Opening mail and paying bills
- Communicating with friends or relatives
- Food preparation
- House cleaning
- Laundry
- Tasks such as taking out the garbage, grass mowing, or snow shoveling

If you agree to take on one or more of these responsibilities, be sure to accept the accountability for doing the task(s), as well. Saying that you will do something and actually doing it are two different matters, and it is too much to expect the primary caregiver to be handing out reminders to other caregivers, or finding last minute replacements for "no shows," in addition to her own caregiving responsibilities.

Helping From Afar

If you do not live in proximity to the dying person, or if your responsibilities prevent you from being a hands on caregiver on a regular basis, you can still be of great assistance to the family members who will be doing the caregiving, and you owe it to them to think of what roles you can assume.

It is important to realize that the primary caregiver is probably stretching herself to the limit to juggle caregiving, work, and/or family responsibilities. Given this, it is reasonable that you will look ahead on your calendar and commit to doing caregiving for a long weekend or a week now and then, even if it requires taking a "red eye" (overnight) flight each way. Doing so will not only give the primary caregiver a few days of respite, but it will open your eyes to the reality of giving care to a seriously ill or dying person. It is very easy, if living afar, to assume that caregiving is a less demanding and less stressful situation than it really is. Taking your turn as a caregiver will correct those misperceptions and make you more grateful for the primary caregiver's sacrifices.

Regardless of the distance you live from the dying person, there are tasks that you can do to relieve the caregiver's burden. For example, you can help with doing internet research on elder service agencies and service providers and then call those service providers to get information concerning their costs and services. You can also be the one to set up a "CaringBridge" web site (see page 159) and/or communicate with other family members and friends via a Facebook page, group email list, or phone tree.

If the primary caregiver does not want to also be attorney-in-fact, perhaps you could take on the role of being attorney-in-fact, setting up an online checking account that you can manage to pay bills (or have payments automatically deducted from the account). Or, if the primary caregiver cannot take the time to draft or revise the will, living will, or other legal documents, you might consider being the one to work with a lawyer to draft new legal documents (NOTE: if you live out of state, make sure that the lawyer that you choose is practicing in the state where your loved one is living, or has passed their State Bar exams and is licensed to practice in the state where your loved one is living! Probate laws vary from state to state, and you do not want to have legal documents that will not be valid in the state in which your loved one resides.)

Respecting, Appreciating, and Supporting the Primary Caregiver

I have a special message for family members and friends who live too far away, or feel that they have too many other responsibilities, to give hands on care on an ongoing basis: If you are not the primary, hands on caregiver, I urge you to respect the efforts of the family member who is doing the daily care with your loved one.

The first aspect of showing respect is not to "second guess" or minimize the primary caregiver's observations and concerns. Unless you are willing to alter your own life by being there in person to take on additional caregiving responsibilities, or move the loved one to be near you so that you are the primary caregiver, the best thing that you can do is to trust the primary caregiver's intentions and not interfere with him doing his duties. It is terribly frustrating for a primary caregiver to have someone at a distance trying to dictate in detail how and when everything should be done.

The second way to show respect is to communicate with the primary caregiver according to his or her preferred method, days, and times. The primary caregiver is already being inconvenienced on a daily basis. It adds unnecessary stress to the caregiver's life to be telephoned at inconvenient hours or to have urgent questions posed by email and then have the sender be upset that the caregiver has not responded, when he has not even had the time to check email in several days.

It is also important to appreciate the primary caregiver and let her know how grateful you are for her efforts. Primary caregivers have lives, too, and just because she lives with or near the dying person doesn't mean that it is easy for her to spend hours a day with an ill person.

Especially if the caregiving period becomes extended for more than a few weeks, family members who are caregivers need to hear your expressions of concern for them and need to know that you are also investing your time—or resources—to improve the caregiving process. The question "What can I do to be helpful?" will be appreciated and will open a dialogue for how you can be a more active participant, even in a less hands on manner.

Finally, if it is possible to do so, having a frank dialogue among family members about roles, responsibilities, and finances can help to address unequal roles among caregivers.

Oftentimes, all of the adult children of a dying person will receive equal shares of whatever estate is left, regardless of how much time each has given, or will give, to caring for the dying person (or his or her spouse). Therefore, it is up to the family members to discuss caregiving inequalities among themselves, to see if a more equitable arrangement can be made, either from the dying person's, or family members', current personal finances, or through redistribution of some of the assets of the estate after the loved one has died.

If the dying person's financial resources are limited, and you as a family member living at a distance (or living locally but unable to assist on a daily basis) have the financial wherewithal to be helpful, consider how your financial contribution can equalize your caregiving role with that of the most involved caregiver. For example, if you are able to finance part-time caregivers so that the primary caregiver can have regular days off, or if you can pay for a short vacation for the primary caregiver, this can enable her to avoid exhaustion or illness and recuperate from the heavy emotional toll that constant caregiving exacts.

CHAPTER FOUR

WHAT DOES IT MEAN TO BE A GOOD CAREGIVER FOR SOMEONE WHO IS DYING?

Taking the "My Wishes" Survey Yourself to Prepare You to Talk With Your Loved One About Her Wishes for End of Life Care

I have designed a "My Wishes" survey that will help you as a caregiver to think about your own preferences, values, likes, and dislikes for your end of life care, so that you can help your dying friend or relative to think about his own preferences, values, likes, and dislikes for her end of life care.

The survey does not ask you to imagine a perfect life, but to reflect on the qualities, activities and other aspects of your life that you enjoy now. The survey then asks you to think about which of those you might want to retain in the final chapter of your life. This survey will also ask you to reflect on any facets of your current life that you may want to leave behind or modify as you decline in health, and which activities or interests you may want to add as time goes on. This sifting process, separating what is desirable and useful now from what may not be desirable or useful when one is dying, is at the core of understanding what it means to live life as fully as possible, and with dignity, until death.

It is fascinating to realize that for any common activity—shopping, cooking, doing yard work, or watching TV, for example—one person will enjoy doing that activity, while another person dislikes that same activity. In other words, we apply our own interpretation as to whether something is enjoyable or distasteful. As caregivers, we cannot assume that our dying spouse, friend, or relative thinks the same way that we do about what activity or situation would be enjoyable, pleasant, annoying, offensive, or distasteful.

I encourage you, in your role as a caregiver, to utilize the "My Wishes" survey to think about your own preferences about what you want in the final stage of your life before reading the survey to your loved one. In this way, you will not be attempting to answer the survey yourself as you are trying to listen carefully and record the thoughts and feelings of the person whom you are assisting.

Keep in mind that flexibility is a key concept in caring for someone and doing it well. Likes and dislikes, as well as abilities, can change from moment to moment, so what your loved one has told you he likes to eat, or wear, or do today may change by tomorrow. The survey is a starting point, not a cast-in-stone plan that cannot be altered. Keeping that in mind, you are now ready to think about what your own wishes are for end of life care.

A "My Wishes" Survey for the Caregiver:

Take a moment to let yourself imagine that you are entering the final chapter of your life, however close or far away from you that may be in reality. In this frame of mind, answer the questions with whatever answers come to you—perhaps from your rational mind, or perhaps from your heart or your "gut sensibility" about how you wish to live your life and be cared for in the final years, months, and days of your life. Don't judge the answer that comes to you. Just write it down, using a pencil, if you wish, so you can change your answers later on.

Activities

a) What activities are (or have been in the past) the most enjoyable, satisfying, or meaningful to you? Be sure to list aspects of work, family life (including pets, if important to you), and hobbies, as well as specific television shows, radio programs, magazines or books, or music that you enjoy.

_____

_____

_____

_____

b) Which of these activities do you want to continue into the final chapter of your life?

_____

_____

_____

c) Are there any new activities that you might want to learn, participate in, or observe?

_____

_____

_____

d) In which activities do you *not* want to participate in the final phase of your life?

_____

_____

_____

e) In which activities do you not even want to be a passive participant, such as watching others?

_____

_____

_____

Values:

What are the values by which you have lived your life? (Some examples of values might be: being a good father/mother/grandparent/guardian; being fair; being the best at (anything that you do); being successful in the work or activity you love; supporting causes you believe in; following your religious principles, telling the truth, or being a loving person.) Do not feel limited by the examples listed above, but use them as a springboard to help you think about your values, as well as the causes you support.

a) What are the values that are important to you and/or causes you have supported or been committed to?

_____

_____

_____

b) Which of these values are most important for you to continue to embody (and which causes do you wish to support) in the last chapter of your life? Are there any new values that you wish to embody or new causes you wish to support?

_____

_____

_____

c) Which values and beliefs should be embodied in your caregivers?

_____

_____

_____

d) Which values and beliefs are contrary to you and which you do *not* want to have embodied in your caregivers?

_____

_____

_____

Physical Environment:

The situations in which people feel comfortable living vary enormously from person to person. Some persons are happiest living in a large home; others are happiest living in a small home. Some persons love lots of decorations; others like simplicity and a lack of decoration.

Some people want to have the constant background sound of a radio or television going throughout the day, or even while sleeping, while others love quiet and want to have a quiet, dark room in which to sleep at night.

Some people have a tendency to overheat, and hence love sleeping in rooms with the windows open or air conditioning on, and only a light blanket. Others never open a window at night and sleep with layers of blankets, except on the warmest of nights.

a) What are the qualities of environment that are most important to you in your current life? (general atmosphere, hot, cold, quiet, music, TV, colors)

_____

_____

b) What qualities of environment do you want most in your final stage of living/dying?

_____

_____

c) What things (furniture, plants, artwork, memorabilia, photographs) or animals (pets) do you want in your environment in your final stage of living and dying?

_____

_____

d) Are there any things (furniture, plants, artwork, memorabilia, photographs) or animals (pets) that you do *not* want in your environment in your final stage of living and dying?

_____

_____

Alone or in Groups?

Some people are natural "extroverts," social beings who like to participate in groups, whether at sports games, NASCAR meets, bingo, concerts, a house of worship, or at the Senior Center.

Other people are naturally "introverts," for whom solitary activities such as reading, or doing crossword puzzles, watching television, or doing a craft alone or with one or two other people are the most delightful activities in the world. For introverts, being alone or with one or two other persons, sharing a walk or conversation or meal, provide an adequate amount of stimulation and companionship.

Understanding your need for aloneness or togetherness is one of the critical questions to ask yourself as you think about choosing the setting in which you wish to spend your final years, months, or days.

a) How much time alone do you currently like to have in your life? How much time with friends or family members do you like to have? How much group time with other people (whom you do not know well) do you like having in your life?

_____

_____

_____

b) How much time alone, time with friends and family, or group time (with others whom you do not know well) do you see yourself needing and wanting in your final phase of life?

_____

_____

_____

c) Do you want your caregivers to be more talkative or quiet in nature? If talkative, what do you want them to talk to you about? Are there specific types of TV or radio programs that you want to watch or listen to?

_____

_____

_____

d) Are there any topics that you do *not* want them to tell you about or discuss with you? Are there any types of radio shows, television programs, or music that you do *not* want them to have on in your presence?

_____

_____

_____

Clothing and Appearance:

Some people are very particular about how they look each day, color coordinating their outfits and wearing matching accessories (and/or make-up or nail polish). They make sure that they change their outfits each day and take particular care about having their clothes pressed and their shoes shined. Other people don't pay much attention to how they look, preferring to wear the same comfortable sweater every day, whether matching their shirt or blouse or not, and wearing few or no accessories (and little or no make-up).

a) What preferences about clothing and appearance are important to you?

_____

_____

_____

b) What would you want caregivers to do for you concerning your clothing and appearance, if you cannot do so for yourself?

_____

_____

_____

c) Do you have favorite items of clothing that you like to wear often? What shoes do you like to wear?

_____

_____

_____

Possessions:

To some people, their possessions are extremely important; to others, physical objects may not be as important. Think about what your relationship is to the things that you have in your life, and answer the following questions:

a. Please list your most important physical possessions here:

_____

_____

_____

_____

b. Please list the objects that you want to have in the room with you in the last months and days of your life. If there are any that you want to have very close by (on your night stand or even in your bed with you) please specify the item and where you want it to be in relation to you:

_____

_____

_____

_____

Personal Care

If you have been in control of most aspects of your life until now, contemplating becoming dependent on others for your personal care may be the hardest thought of all. For many people, learning to ask for and accept helping in bathing, dressing and undressing, and using the toilet is the greatest challenge in their later years. Yet, the process of becoming increasingly dependent on others can honor your wishes for independence, maintain your dignity, and respect your capacities and limitations as well as those of the people you love, if you communicate your wishes regarding these matters.

a) What are the personal care routines that you want to do for yourself, as long as you can possibly do so?

_____

_____

_____

_____

b) What are specific personal care routines that you wish to have done by a family member (name_____) or close friend (name_____) if at all possible, rather than by a paid caregiver:

_____

_____

_____

c) How often and when do you brush your teeth? If you have dentures, where are they kept? If you floss your teeth, how regularly do you floss them?

_____

_____

_____

Other preferences, wishes and notes regarding personal care:

_____

_____

_____

Religion and Spirituality:

a) Are you a member of a particular religion? Do you attend a particular house of worship? If so, which one:

_____

b) If you are no longer a member of a house of worship, is there a particular religion with which you identify?

_____

c) Is there a particular clergyperson whom you would like to visit you while you are ill or while you are dying?

_____

c) Are there any writings of a spiritual or religious nature that you would want someone to read to you when you are no longer able to ask them to do so?

_____

d) Is there any particular music that is important or sacred to you that you would want played in your final days and hours?

_____

_____

Your final days and hours:

a. If you had the choice, would you rather live out your last days:

_____ In your own home

_____ In the home of someone else: _____

_____ In a live-in hospice care center

_____ In a nursing home with hospice care

_____ In a nursing home without hospice care

Other place:

_____

b. Who are the people that you most want to have around you in the last days and hours of your life?

_____

c. Are there any people whom you do NOT want to have around you when you are in the last phase of your life?

_____

d. If given the chance, would you want to be alone when you die? _____

Would you like to have someone with you when you die?_____
If you wish to have a person or persons with you as you die, please list their names here:

_____

_____

Anything Else?

Is there any family matter (or family secret) that you want us to know about? Is there anything that you need to do for someone or say to someone before you leave this earth in order to leave with a clear conscience? (You do not need to give the details here, unless you want to; if you want us to locate someone from your past or make sure that you talk to someone while you can still do so, please let me know their name and any contact information you may have about them, so we can honor your wishes.)

_____

_____

_____

Is anything else that you want to tell me regarding what honoring your wishes in the last phase of your life means to you?

_____

_____

_____

_____

_____

_____

Using the "My Wishes" Survey to Talk to Your Loved One About Their Wishes for End of Life Care

Now that you as a caregiver (or future caregiver) have done this exercise yourself and written your own thoughts down, you can better help someone else think about these questions for themselves.

If your loved one doesn't want to talk to you about end of life care because he is in denial about dying at all, or if she is no longer able to communicate with you, you can talk with your loved one's spouse, siblings, friends, or neighbors to seek answers to these questions (for example, what clothing did he usually wear when you had coffee with him in the morning? Was it always the same shirt or sweater or was his outfit always different? What was his favorite chair to sit in? Did he tell you any special stories? Did he mention specific items in his house as being important?)

(NOTE: you should feel free to omit or modify questions that are not appropriate for the person who is dying, given their particular health status, mental health status, or other factors)

Activities

a) What activities are (or have been in the past) the most enjoyable, satisfying, or meaningful to you? Be sure to list aspects of work, family life (including pets, if important to you), and hobbies, as well as specific television shows, radio programs, magazines or books, or music that you enjoy.

_____

_____

_____

_____

b) Which of these activities do you want to continue into the final chapter of your life?

_____

_____

_____

c) Are there any new activities that you might want to learn, participate in, or observe?

_____

_____

_____

d) In which activities do you *not* want to participate in the final phase of your life?

_____

_____

_____

e) In which activities do you not even want to be a passive participant, such as watching others?

_____

_____

_____

Values:

What are the values by which you have lived your life? (Some examples of values might be: being a good father/mother/grandparent/guardian; being fair; being the best at (anything that you do); being successful in the work or activity you love; supporting causes you believe in; following your religious principles, telling the truth, or being a loving person.) Do not feel limited by the examples listed above, but use them as a springboard to help you think about your values, as well as the causes you support.

a) What are the values that are important to you and/or causes you have supported or been committed to?

_____

_____

_____

b) Which of these values are most important for you to continue to embody (and which causes do you wish to support) in the last chapter of your life? Are there any new values that you wish to embody or new causes you wish to support?

_____

_____

_____

c) Which values and beliefs should be embodied in your caregivers?

_____

_____

_____

d) Which values and beliefs are contrary to you and which you do *not* want to have embodied in your caregivers?

_____

_____

_____

Physical Environment:

The situations in which people feel comfortable living vary enormously from person to person. Some persons are happiest living in a large home; others are happiest living in a small home. Some persons love lots of decorations; others like simplicity and a lack of decoration.

Some people want to have the constant background sound of a radio or television going throughout the day, or even while sleeping, while others love quiet and want to have a quiet, dark room in which to sleep at night.

Some people have a tendency to overheat, and hence love sleeping in rooms with the windows open or air conditioning on, and only a light blanket. Others never open a window at night and sleep with layers of blankets, except on the warmest of nights.

a) What are the qualities of environment that are most important to you in your current life? (general atmosphere, hot, cold, quiet, music, TV, colors)

_____

_____

b) What qualities of environment do you want most in your final stage of living/dying?

_____

_____

c) What things (furniture, plants, artwork, memorabilia, photographs) or animals (pets) do you want in your environment in your final stage of living and dying?

_____

_____

d) Are there any things (furniture, plants, artwork, memorabilia, photographs) or animals (pets) that you do *not* want in your environment in your final stage of living and dying?

_____

_____

Alone or in Groups?

Some people are natural "extroverts," social beings who like to participate in groups, whether at sports games, NASCAR meets, bingo, concerts, a house of worship, or at the Senior Center.

Other people are naturally "introverts," for whom solitary activities such as reading, or doing crossword puzzles, watching television, or doing a craft alone or with one or two other people are the most delightful activities in the world. For introverts, being alone or with one or two other persons, sharing a walk or conversation or meal, provide an adequate amount of stimulation and companionship.

Understanding your need for aloneness or togetherness is one of the critical questions to ask yourself as you think about choosing the setting in which you wish to spend your final years, months, or days.

a) How much time alone do you currently like to have in your life? How much time with friends or family members do you like to have? How much group time with other people (whom you do not know well) do you like having in your life?

_____

_____

_____

b) How much time alone, time with friends and family, or group time (with others whom you do not know well) do you see yourself needing and wanting in your final phase of life?

_____

_____

_____

c) Do you want your caregivers to be more talkative or quiet in nature? If talkative, what do you want them to talk to you about? Are there specific types of TV or radio programs that you want to watch or listen to?

_____

_____

_____

d) Are there any topics that you do *not* want them to tell you about or discuss with you? Are there any types of radio shows, television programs, or music that you do *not* want them to have on in your presence?

_____

_____

_____

Clothing and Appearance:

Some people are very particular about how they look each day, color coordinating their outfits and wearing matching accessories (and/or make-up or nail polish). They make sure that they change their outfits each day and take particular care about having their clothes pressed and their shoes shined. Other people don't pay much attention to how they look, preferring to wear the same comfortable sweater every day, whether matching their shirt or blouse or not, and wearing few or no accessories (and little or no make-up).

a) What preferences about clothing and appearance are important to you?

_____

_____

_____

b) What would you want caregivers to do for you concerning your clothing and appearance, if you cannot do so for yourself?

_____

_____

_____

c) Do you have favorite items of clothing that you like to wear often? What shoes do you like to wear?

_____

_____

_____

Possessions:

To some people, their possessions are extremely important; to others, physical objects may not be as important. Think about what your relationship is to the things that you have in your life, and answer the following questions:

a. Please list your most important physical possessions here:

_____

_____

_____

_____

b. Please list the objects that you want to have in the room with you in the last months and days of your life. If there are any that you want to have very close by (on your night stand or even in your bed with you) please specify the item and where you want it to be in relation to you:

_____

_____

_____

_____

Personal Care

If you have been in control of most aspects of your life until now, contemplating becoming dependent on others for your personal care may be the hardest thought of all. For many people, learning to ask for and accept helping in bathing, dressing and undressing, and using the toilet is the greatest challenge in their later years. Yet, the process of becoming increasingly dependent on others can honor your wishes for independence, maintain your dignity, and respect your capacities and limitations as well as those of the people you love, if you communicate your wishes regarding these matters.

a) What are the personal care routines that you want to do for yourself, as long as you can possibly do so?

_____

_____

_____

_____

b) What are specific personal care routines that you wish to have done by a family member (name_____) or close friend (name_____) if at all possible, rather than by a paid caregiver:

_____

_____

_____

c) How often and when do you brush your teeth? If you have dentures, where are they kept? If you floss your teeth, how regularly do you floss them?

_____

_____

_____

Other preferences, wishes and notes regarding personal care:

_____

_____

_____

Religion and Spirituality:

a) Are you a member of a particular religion? Do you attend a particular house of worship? If so, which one:

_____

b) If you are no longer a member of a house of worship, is there a particular religion with which you identify?

_____

c) Is there a particular clergyperson whom you would like to visit you while you are ill or while you are dying?

_____

c) Are there any writings of a spiritual or religious nature that you would want someone to read to you when you are no longer able to ask them to do so?

_____

d) Is there any particular music that is important or sacred to you that you would want played in your final days and hours?

_____

_____

Your final days and hours:

a. If you had the choice, would you rather live out your last days:

____ In your own home

____ In the home of someone else: _____

____ In a live-in hospice care center

____ In a nursing home with hospice care

____ In a nursing home without hospice care

Other place:

_____

b. Who are the people that you most want to have around you in the last days and hours of your life?

_____

c. Are there any people whom you do NOT want to have around you when you are in the last phase of your life?

_____

d. If given the chance, would you want to be alone when you die? _____

Would you like to have someone with you when you die?_____
If you wish to have a person or persons with you as you die, please list their names here:

_____

_____

Anything Else?

Is there any family matter (or family secret) that you want us to know about? Is there anything that you need to do for someone or say to someone before you leave this earth in order to leave with a clear conscience? (You do not need to give the details here, unless you want to; if you want us to locate someone from your past or make sure that you talk to someone while you can still do so, please let me know their name and any contact information you may have about them, so we can honor your wishes.)

_____

_____

_____

Is anything else that you want to tell me regarding what honoring your wishes in the last phase of your life means to you?

_____

_____

_____

_____

_____

_____

CHAPTER FIVE

COMMUNICATION

- Family Meeting
- Doing an Intervention
- Devising a "Plan B"
- Communication Tools: CaringBridge, Email Lists, and Other Ways to Stay in Touch
- Dealing with Family Difficulties
- When Conflicts Cannot Be Resolved
- Finding Your Own North Star

I stated in the first chapter something that bears repeating, namely that when I use the term family, I do not mean to imply that families have any particular configuration or that family members must be biologically related. Families can be biological or they can be "chosen," including persons who are friends, business associates, church or temple members, or any others who function as family, whether or not they are related by blood or marriage.

Family Meeting

I encourage you to communicate with other family members about your own wishes and their wishes for caring for your loved one at the end of his or her life, rather than assuming that they will agree with what you think the plan should be. The final stage of caring for a dying person can bring to the surface surprisingly different—and emotionally charged—viewpoints among family members. It is better to find out where the differences are before you have to make split-second decisions in a crisis. This is where a family meeting comes into the picture.

Having a face-to-face family meeting is far superior to telephone conference calls or even Skype video-phone conversations when it comes to making important decisions. Even if some family members live far away, it is worth making every attempt to have a face-to-face meeting with family members, to establish a "game plan" and secure people's commitments to that plan.

One of the most major decisions that needs to be made is where to care for the dying person. Some family members may want to have the dying person stay in his home, but others may want to move the dying person to a nursing facility. If this deep rift in viewpoints becomes apparent, you will want to be together, face to face, to talk about this important issue.

If members of the family are not willing to inconvenience themselves to attend and participate in such a meeting, then they should also be willing to relinquish their voting power concerning important decisions that need to be made. There is nothing helpful about having absentee family members not be willing to modify their schedules or expend their resources, yet feel entitled to ignore concerns of the primary caregiver or override his recommendations about what to do or not do.

If your disagreements cannot be solved, there are several options to consider, depending on the particular family structure you have and the circumstances before you.

Doing an Intervention

When my grandmother was failing in health, two of her grown children wanted to move her to a nursing home. The other grown child was opposed to the plan, but was outvoted and felt powerless to do anything about it. Upon hearing of this plan, several of us grandchildren collaborated to see if we could block the attempt to move her to a nursing home and allow her to die at home under hospice care.

One of us contacted the social worker of the hospice that was providing her care and discussed our concerns and our desires to keep her in the home where she had lived for forty years. After sharing our feelings about this issue and discussing possible steps to take, the social worker agreed to support us in holding an "intervention," a meeting at the grandmother's house to which as many of us grown grandchildren as possible would come at a specified time, parking our vehicles away from the home.

The grown child who had proposed moving our grandmother to a nursing home was then invited to come to the grandmother's home. That elder was met by a room of adult grandchildren who said, in no uncertain terms, that our grandmother would not be moved to a nursing home. The social worker was there to talk about the practicalities of at home hospice care and to secure our commitment as a family to being responsible for her care. I became the hospice care coordinator and one of her primary caregivers. I am glad to say that our grandmother lived the last three months of her life exactly as she wanted to live them—in her own home, in her bedroom, with its wonderful flowered wallpaper and tall antique dressers, with the light streaming through the large windows, and her pink magnolia tree and purple irises visible through those windows.

Devising a "Plan B"

Such interventions are not always possible. A friend of mine had a similar situation develop, but with a different outcome. Her siblings made the decision to move their mother to a nursing home rather than caring for her in her own home. Without a sufficient number of family members willing to offer hands on support, and without adequate financial resources, she was unable to affect the decision.

She enlisted the help of a psychotherapist, not to do an intervention, but to work on her own personal conflicts and emotions and come up with a workable "Plan B." The therapist assured her that conflicts within families concerning end of life issues are very common, and that often one person with a minority position cannot sway the outcome. Through counseling, she realized that she could do nothing to change the decision to move her mother to the nursing home.

However, she came to realize that she could still fulfill a promise that she had made to her father as he was dying several years earlier— to provide the best possible care to her mother after his death— regardless of where her mother would spend her last years and months. She also accepted the fact that this would mean visiting and caring for her mother on a daily basis, since problems kept surfacing at the nursing care facility and her siblings were not willing to establish any schedule regarding when they would visit. Thus, rather than feeling powerless to affect an outcome that she did not choose, she was able to implement "Plan B," which enabled her to meet her personal commitments and goals for her mother's care, regardless of the decision to move their mother from her home to an institutional care facility.

Communication Tools: CaringBridge, Email Lists, and Other Ways to Stay in Touch

In the years in which this book was being written, new communications tools have come into being, and these are a great boon to families who are dealing with caring for a loved one.

One of the most innovative technologies via the Internet is called **CaringBridge** (www.caringbridge.org). CaringBridge is a nonprofit organization that provides confidential, easy to use websites for families or groups that are seeking to support a loved one with acute or chronic medical problems and who wish to stay in touch with each other. The web templates are easy to launch, and require no knowledge of special computer languages.

Facebook (www.facebook.com) is another web-based technology where a family group or individual can set up a web page and then communicate with only family members or make information available on a more expanded basis.

Skype (www.skype.com) is a web-based telecommunications tool that allows both voice and images to be sent via an internet connection. With the use of a "webcam" (web camera) which can be plugged into either a laptop or desk top computer, and the downloading of free Skype software, it is now possible to see your loved one or loved ones while talking on the phone.

Twitter and texting are the preferred methods of communication for the younger set. The ever-increasing millions of persons using text-based technologies via cell phone, Blackberry, and I Phones show me that these will probably overshadow my favorite method of communicating with friends, **email,** the older "texting" technology. There are useful characteristics about email: it allows the author to send a much longer message than via Twitter, and a large number of addresses can be put into a group email list so that one message can be sent to all members, and the reply can be received by all members.

Communication notebooks (spiral bound, lined one-subject books are inexpensive and work well) are the oldest communication tool, but are still very valuable. If you are caring for your loved one at home, and only with family members and friends as caregivers, you probably need only one notebook. I have found it helpful, when paid caregivers from an agency are involved, to have a separate notebook (make sure it has a different color cover and is clearly labeled) for notes to and from the paid caregiver (the caregiver's full name, date and time of arrival and departure, and notes from them about what they did and observed, or any questions that they have; and notes with name, date and time, and comment or question from the family member to the caregiver.) The notebook for the family can include stories of a more personal nature ("Mom was speaking to Dad tonight as if he were still alive" or questions for family members "Can someone buy more Oil of Olay for Mom in the next week?")

If your loved one is in a nursing facility or hospital, you will need only the family notebook, and you should buy one of the smaller variety (6 by 9 inches or so) because space is at a premium and you want to be able to tuck the family notebook in a bedside table or dresser drawer, rather than leaving it out.

Whether you prefer to communicate in writing, or via phone, email, or web-based communications tools, you will be able to set up ways to communicate that are much easier to use than those that existed only a decade ago. Since new technologies are being developed every day, I invite you to checkout my website, www.caringfordyinglovedones.com, where I will post information on the latest ways for families to communicate with each other.

Dealing with Family Difficulties

What I have come to understand over time, through caring for loved ones and talking to friends who have also done the same, is that oftentimes one family member will take on the primary responsibility of being the ongoing caregiver, while others are much less involved, perhaps visiting every week or two, or even far less often. This difference in responsibility level may be a result of persons living farther from the dying person, from the fact that others feel unable to emotionally deal with the situation, because they have (or feel they have) other commitments that prevent their involvement, or because the family member's spouse or partner may not support them giving the time to the dying person.

Differences in caregiving attitudes, responsibilities, and frequency of caregiving can create difficult feelings between family members. Sometimes these difficulties can be resolved through dialogue or professionally facilitated meetings, and sometimes the best solution is simply to wait until the loved one has died, and let time heal the emotional strain on the relationships. After a period of time has passed, it may be possible to accept that each person did the best that they could, even though it was not sufficient to meet your needs, or your loved one's needs, at the time.

When Conflicts Cannot Be Resolved

There are family situations in which conflicts are so deep, and so complex, that they cause permanent rifts between family members. If you find yourself in such a situation, I encourage you to seek professional help to come to terms with your own anger, sadness, or other emotions. Even if healing the rift with the other family member is impossible to do, professional counsel may assist you in finding a way to deal with your emotions so that you do not feel stuck in the past, reliving past painful encounters.

I have found that a psychotherapeutic technique called EMDR, which stands for Eye Movement Desensitization and Reprocessing, has been very helpful in dealing with difficult experiences from my past. EMDR is a short-term psychotherapy technique, one that, in my own layperson's terms, can take traumatic or unresolved issues and "put a clear bubble around them," so that they do not spontaneously "trigger" strong emotions and difficult memories in daily life. To find out about EMDR, please see the listing under EMDR on page 160 in the resource section of this book.

Finding Your Own North Star

The "north star" by which I steered my ship in caring for my mother was continually asking myself what I wanted to do to live out my values and care for my loved one to the best of my ability. Looking back on the final two years of my caring for her, I would do some things differently if I had them to do over again, but in each instance I did the best possible job that I could do at that time.

Two years after my mother's passing, I feel a deep sense of gratitude for all that happened, the good times as well as the difficulties, and I know that I would take on that primary caregiving role again if I were to have the chance to relive this chapter in my life.

Each person in a family will need to decide for him or herself what role they will play in this process of helping the dying person. The answers may be very different and these differences may place you in opposition to your loved ones, but if you decide rightly for yourself, being true to yourself will have its own reward.

This is the goal in choosing your own path as a caregiver—to be able to look back on the days, months, or years of caregiving—no matter how challenging—and to be able to know in your heart that you did what was right for you in service of your loved one.

CHAPTER SIX

THE "DO IT NOW" LIST

- Health Care Proxy and Living Will
- Sample Living Will Language
- HIPAA (Rules for Disclosure of Medical Records)
- Will
- Durable Power of Attorney
- Creating a List of Relatives and Friends
- Writing an Obituary
- Obituary Draft Form
- Burial, Cremation, Funeral, Visiting Hours, Memorial Service
- Religious Tradition and House of Worship
- Pre-Arranging Funeral Services
- Funeral Planning Checklist
- Cemetery Burials and Green Burials; Burying or Scattering Ashes
- Veterans' Benefits
- Headstone
- Social Security Benefits
- Personalizing Memorial Services
- Reception

Ideally, each of us would have all the time we need to think about what our wishes are for our end of life care and have enough time to communicate that to those whom we love. For some, the luxury of time for extended reflection is not available. If your loved one has suffered a catastrophic accident, or if she has had a massive stroke or another illness that has rendered her in urgent need of care, the practical aspects of caring for your loved one must be dealt with immediately. Each person's situation is unique, so you will need to decide which of the items listed here to do first, second, and third.

The most important thing to keep in mind as you decide which items are of greatest importance to you is that the dying person may lose all ability to communicate, either through voice, writing, pointing, head-shaking, or even blinking her eyes at some point in her dying process. This loss of ability to communicate may come suddenly, with no warning, and may happen well in advance of actually dying.

The loss of ability to communicate with my loved ones was the most difficult challenge for me as a caregiver. My recognition of this has prompted me to highlight the activities and tasks below that require communication with the person who is dying. The loss of a relative's or friend's ability to communicate will forever remove the opportunity to discuss, share, exchange, and relay important information, *so please do not take your communication with your loved one for granted!* I hope that you will review the list below and decide to discuss these important items with your loved one at the earliest appropriate time. Please do not assume that handling the important tasks mentioned below can wait until another day.

The Health Care Proxy and Living Will

Writing (or updating) the person's health care proxy (the document naming the person who will be health care agent) and the living will (medical directive).

The importance of the medical directive, detailing the person's desire for care in acute illness and when dying cannot be over stated. This is the chance for the dying person to articulate what her wishes are for the kind of medical care she will receive and to name the person who should make medical decisions for her if she is not capable of doing so.

Most states have their own Health Care Proxy form. It can be helpful, but is not necessary, to consult with a lawyer before filling it out. Most physicians' offices and all hospitals can supply copies of the form. However, be aware that in hospitals, the case managers, social services, or social workers' office may be the place to find that form, and often those offices are not open in the evening or overnight hours! *I found this out firsthand when I accompanied an elderly friend to the emergency room in the middle of the night after she had fallen and broken a hip. I had to go home and go online to my state government's web site to download a copy of the Health Care Proxy form in order to bring it to the hospital.* It is good to know that you can do this, if you need a Health Care Proxy form and cannot get one from a doctor's office or from a case manager at the hospital during normal business hours. (Better yet, go your state's web site and print out a copy of the form before you urgently need it!)

Note: it is a good idea for all people, not just dying people, to have copies of their Health Care Proxy form and medical directive filed with their doctor, with their health care agent and alternate agent, put into a "File of Life" packet on the refrigerator door, and also keep a copy with themselves at all times. None of us is immune from sudden accidents, and carrying a Health Care Proxy form will inform emergency personnel to contact the health care agent if you are not capable of making your own medical decisions.

Choosing the person to communicate with physicians concerning the dying person's care, if she or he can no longer do so, is a very important matter. It is my recommendation that you talk with the dying person about his choices for end of life medical care and have him write out his/her wishes (or initial the choices on pages 167–172) before having the dying person decide who should be his health care agent. The dying person (or you) should then discuss his wishes for end of life care with the person(s) he is thinking of choosing as the health care agent and alternate agent, to ensure that the chosen health care agent and alternate agent are in agreement with the dying person's wishes and can make a commitment to upholding their wishes. Simply assuming that the agent holds the same values as the dying person will not guarantee that his wishes will be fulfilled.

To illustrate this point, let me relay a story about a friend of mine. This friend had told me on many occasions that she wanted to die at home and did not want to spend even one day in a nursing home, especially if she was totally dependent on others for care, such as being in diapers and unable to walk or feed or dress herself. However, she did not specifically speak to her health care agent about these end of life wishes, nor did she articulate them in such detail in her medical directive, except to say that she did not want to be resuscitated if her heart failed and did not want to have her life prolonged if she were in a vegetative state.

My friend experienced a massive stroke that removed her ability to speak, write, point to pictures, or even shake her head or blink her eyes in response to questions. Her health care agent, unaware of the friend's feelings about not wanting to go to a nursing home, was advised by doctors not to let her go home from the hospital (even though she could have afforded at home care) but to bring her to a nursing home "until she grew stronger."

Because she had suffered a massive stroke, once in the nursing home, she was labeled a "fall risk" and was confined to a wheelchair via a tether and an alarm, except for brief periods of physical therapy each day. This restriction, supposedly done out of concern for her safety (but done as much for the sake of the nursing home's liability) took away any opportunity for her to stand, walk, and grow stronger. Her anger at being tethered to the wheel chair (and to being in the nursing home in diapers) was constantly evident in her exasperated sighs and her attempts to push her wheelchair through alarmed exit doors, even though she had no ability to speak.

Her physical resistance to being put into the wheelchair each day, and her attempts to wheel herself through the emergency exit doors, were interpreted by the medical staff as a psychiatric disorder. She was given increased levels of psychiatric medications that diminished her personality, her spirit, and her will to live. She died within a few months of her stroke, never having had the chance to return to her own apartment.

Having observed this sad scenario, I have now revised my medical directive to be much more specific as to my wishes for end of life care, not only concerning "vegetative state" conditions (which are the usual ones mentioned in living wills), but the more common debilitations of stroke, heart disease, dementia, and chronic illness.

Sample Living Will Language

Using a website search engine such as Google.com brings up many pages concerning health care directives (living wills). I suggest that you read the language in different directives before deciding on the final language for your own, or your loved one's, directive. **Please see page 163 under Living Will for a web site to consult, and appendices A and B (pages 167–172)** for sample wording that you may wish to use in creating a Medical Directive (Living Will). This document can be worded in any way to address the needs and concerns of your loved one. The important thing is that your loved one has the opportunity to express his wishes concerning end of life care, and that those wishes be communicated to the health care agent and alternate agent, family members, the physician or physicians, and any persons, paid or unpaid, who may be involved in the dying person's care.

NOTE: The person whom you choose to carry out your wishes for end of life care should be someone with a strong sense of integrity and someone who will fight for your wishes, even if others in the family (or, perhaps, medical providers) attempt to block those wishes based on their different values, wishes, or religious beliefs.

A friend of mine told me, "I did not understand why the physician who was caring for my loved one kept saying that he did not qualify for end of life hospice care, even though all signs told me that he was dying. I learned, through talking to various people, that this physician didn't believe in hospice care. This information made me realize that we would have to take action on our own to have him admitted to hospice care."

If the physician caring for your loved one resists talking about admission to hospice, ask him if he has admitted patients to hospice before, and which hospice he has worked with. This may alert you to the fact that the physician considers "admission to hospice" to be "admission of failure" on his part. In this case, contact the hospice directly to see about getting a consultation by another physician.

The issue of integrity is also important when the person who is designated as the health care agent will receive any portion of the dying person's estate. While all of us would like to think that someone whom we trusted would make decisions about our medical care with our best interest in mind, the person who does not have a strong commitment to integrity might not honor the dying person's wishes if deciding on a less expensive treatment option would preserve more of the assets of the estate and personally benefit him in the long run.

HIPAA

The federal Health Insurance Portability and Accountability Act of 1996 (HIPAA) created rules to protect the privacy of a patient's medical record. For a health care agent, alternate agent, and others to have access to a loved one's medical record, the HIPAA release authorization should be included in the health care proxy or the HIPAA authorization form should be completed and made effective immediately. Do not wait until a crisis to complete this document. (See page 162)

Will

If the dying person already has a will, now is the time to find it and for her to review it and make any necessary revisions. If the person does not already have a will, now is the time to help her in writing one.

Since probate laws vary by state, I recommend seeking the professional assistance of an attorney in the state where your loved one resides as the best method for having legal documents that will be done correctly and stand up to scrutiny, should they be contested in court.

The cost of hiring an attorney to write the will and power of attorney documents can range from as little as $100 to $2,000 or more depending on the complexity of the estate and the experience and location of the attorney. If you have limited or no income, you can contact your state bar association to ask if you can be referred to a lawyer who will work on a pro bono (free) or reduced fee basis. Another low cost option is that in some locations, lawyers offer low cost methods of doing simple wills and power of attorney documents for groups of individuals. In this scenario, the lawyer sends a packet of information to the individuals, and each fills out a template form regarding their wishes. Then, 15 or so individuals bring their forms to a presentation about wills and power of attorney documents. After the presentation, lawyers review each person's template documents in a brief, confidential meeting, at which time revisions can be made. Each person is able to leave with a notarized simple will and a power of attorney document.

Whether you see a lawyer as an individual or family, or you attend a group presentation followed by a confidential meeting with a lawyer, I encourage you to consult a lawyer to draft these documents so that the person's intentions are clear according to the probate laws of the state in which he or she lives.

However, if you wish to look into online templates for wills and powers of attorney, I suggest visiting www.nolo.com first, for it is a reputable organization that was founded in 1971 to educate the public about the law. Nolo.com offers a variety of free and low-cost legal resources, concerning wills, trusts, tenant-landlord matters, contracts, and many other legal matters.

Durable Power of Attorney

The Durable Power of Attorney names the attorney-in-fact, the person designated to carry on financial affairs if the dying person is not capable of doing so. (The word "Durable" is very important, for it means that the document will continue to be in effect even after the person has lost capacity.) If the dying person already has a Durable Power of Attorney document, now is the time for him or her to review it and have a lawyer make any necessary revisions. If the person does not already have a Durable Power of Attorney document, now is the time to have one drafted by a lawyer. Many attorneys advise making the document effective immediately, even if a person is not yet extremely ill, so that someone can handle their affairs, if needed. (Persons who are well but who will be traveling for any length of time may also want to activate their Power of Attorney document so that others can handle their affairs in their absence.)

Note: if a lawyer, accountant, or other professional service provider is named to be someone's attorney-in-fact, they will be able to charge their hourly rate (which could be $300 an hour, or more) for every quarter-hour of work done for the dying person, including paying regular bills and communicating with family members. Unless there is a complicated estate, or no one from the family is able to assume the responsibility of the power of attorney, it will protect the assets of the estate to have a family member take on this responsibility, rather than naming a lawyer or accountant. The family member can be reimbursed for their time at a much lower rate per hour, or she may do this work on a voluntary basis.

Creating a List of Relatives and Friends

If you are lucky, you will still be able to ask the dying person "Who are the most important people in your life right now? Who comes to visit you? Who calls you? Who writes to you?" If you have been living far from the dying person, you may not have any idea that the man living two houses up from your father comes to have coffee every morning with him, or that your mother's old childhood friend calls once a week to talk on the phone. Be sure to ask your loved one who the people are who call or visit, and how often, to get a sense of who his or her closest friends really are.

Even if your loved one cannot talk to you, see if you can find an address book, a holiday card list, a perpetual calendar, a cell phone (or an older phone with a memory function) or a Rolodex that you can use as a starting point for this list. If not, you can create a list from scratch, starting from the closest family members (in relation and proximity) and then moving to widening concentric circles of more distant relatives and friends. Begin your list by writing down a title for the list, such as Friends and Family of [the dying person's formal name, as well as their nickname].

Then, write on each line the name, address, city/state, zip and phone number(s) of the friend or relative. If you do not have a full address for each family member or friend, the name and state are the most basic pieces of information needed to do an internet search via www.whitepages.com, www.zabasearch.com, www.anywho.com, www.dogpile.com, www.peoplefinders.com, or other internet search engines. Be sure to compare several internet searches. Doing so can often yield the full address, phone number, email address, and relatives living with the person, if the person's full name, city/state, and approximate age are known.

One caveat: search engine information can be accurate or very outdated. There can also be several listings for the same person, one of which is current and the others of which are inaccurate. If you find several listings, copy down all of them, because you may need to call each number before finding out which is the correct one.

It may also be helpful to have a few close relatives or friends of the dying person review the lists that you have or supply information to you concerning other relatives or friends and their contact information.

If it is still possible to do so, talk to the dying person about what kind of communication she wants to have with each person before her death. I have found it helpful to put the legend **"Visit"** next to the names of persons he/or she would like to have come visit before the person dies, **"Call"** for those with whom she/he wishes to speak by phone, or **"Mail** (or **Email**)"** for those who should be contacted via mail or email prior to the person's death. **"Inform"** is the legend I use for those who should only be informed *after* the person's death. (I put an **"X"** next to the names of those for whom no contact should be/need be made, and **"Deceased"** in front of the name, if the friend or relative has died.)

The goal is to determine who the most important people are and to put some legend next to those names to indicate the dying person's wishes for how to communicate with them. The dying person may or may not wish to receive many visitors as they become more ill. This is their time to tell you their wishes so that you can invite the most important persons to come and say what they need to say or simply sit quietly and silently express their good-byes.

List of important persons (attach additional lists, if needed):

_____

_____

_____

_____

_____

_____

_____

_____

_____

_____

_____

_____

_____

_____

_____

_____

_____

_____

_____

_____

_____

_____

_____

Writing an Obituary

If your loved one has not already written his own obituary, ask him if he wishes to write one or help you write one. If he does not want to think about writing an obituary, you can incorporate questions from the form below into your conversations to elicit the information that will allow you to write an obituary for him.

Many newspapers have increased their cost per word of paid death notices (obituaries) in the past few years, to help offset the loss of advertising revenue. An obituary can cost hundreds of dollars for a modest (four inch long) paid death notice in a local newspaper, and the costs are even greater for urban newspapers and those with regional or national distribution. Be sure to ask the funeral director about the rate per word for the newspaper in which you want the obituary to run before submitting the obituary to the funeral director if you wish to work within a specific budget for the obituary.

Be sure to state explicitly in any funeral contracts that are drawn up that the funeral director will submit the obituary or obituaries to newspapers.

I had an unfortunate experience that illustrates what can happen if this is not made clear: I had not seen an explicit statement concerning the funeral director submitting the obituary in the funeral plans that I had made with the funeral home six months prior to my mother's death, but it didn't concern me since the same funeral home had taken care of this task after my father had died. I was shocked to be told by the funeral director on the morning of my mother's death that "it would be best for me to submit the obituaries to the local papers." When I questioned him about this, he simply stated once more that it would be best if I did this. To add to the stress of this situation, when I called the funeral director on the phone from my home with questions regarding photo file formats or deadlines for submission, he said that he didn't have the information that I needed.

In the midst of my despair at having lost my mother, I had to make multiple telephone calls and leave voice messages at two newspapers in order to reach the appropriate person at each paper and submit the obituary by the late afternoon deadline. This was an incredibly stressful situation for me, and I consider this to have been a professional lapse of responsibility on that funeral director's part.

Obituary Draft Form for:

NAME:_____

Where were you born? (city, state, country)_____

_____

What is your date of birth?_____

What are/were your parents', step-parents', or guardians' names?

Father: (first, middle, last, suffix):_____

Deceased?___ Yr. ___

Father's nickname (if used): _____

Mother: (first, middle, last suffix): _____

Deceased?___ Yr. ___

Mother's maiden name: _____

Mother's nickname (if used): _____

Other close relatives names/relationships:

_____Deceased?____Yr. ___

_____Deceased?____Yr. ___

_____Deceased?____Yr. ___

_____Deceased?____Yr. ___

_____Deceased?____Yr. ___

_____Deceased?____Yr. ___

_____Deceased?____Yr. ___

_____Deceased?____Yr. ___

_____Deceased?____Yr. ___

Pet(s) name(s) (if desired to include):

_____

_____

Where did you grow up?_____

What schools did you attend (this could be elementary, junior high, high school, college, graduate school, or technical schools):

School or college   Years attended   Diploma or Degree Received

_____

_____

_____

_____

Where did you work?
(Start with most recent, and work back from there)

Company/Organization   City/State   Position   Years

_____

_____

_____

_____

_____

_____

_____

Are you, or were you, a member of any fraternal, nonprofit, or religious groups or societies? If so, which ones and where, and did you hold any offices or serve on any committees?

Organization/ position and/or committee:

_____

_____

_____

_____

Did you receive any honors or awards? (Skip if not relevant)

_____

_____

What hobbies, activities, or interests have you had outside of work?

_____

_____

_____

_____

What do you think of as your greatest accomplishments in your life?
What are you most proud of in your life?

_____

_____

_____

_____

Are you a member of a religion?_____

Are you a member of a particular house of worship?

_____

Do you know the name of a particular clergyperson there?

_____

Names of other relatives or friends:
Name   Relationship   City/State   Deceased Y/N (and yr if known)

_____

_____

_____

_____

_____

_____

What photo of yourself do you like the most (and would want used for an obituary or in a memorial program)?

Description   Where can photo be found?

_____

Would you like to print a special statement of thanks to caregivers or others?

_____

_____

_____

_____

Do you want to print a statement of "in lieu of flowers, people may contribute to [cause or causes]"?

Organization or Cause (Complete mailing address, including zip code)

_____

_____

_____

In which newspaper(s) would you want me to print an obituary?

_____

Do you wish to have the obituary submitted to a newspaper in another city or town, as well as this newspaper? To alumni magazines or newsletters?

Newspaper/alumni magazine/newsletter   City/state

_____

_____

_____

_____

_____

Have you prearranged your funeral? ___

If so, where?_____

(If you have made funeral arrangements, have you pre-paid for them?_____)

Other information to be included in an obituary:
Funeral home to handle arrangements:

_____

Street address, city, state   Telephone number   Website

_____

_____

Wake/Shiva: _____

Memorial Service: _____

Religious Service: _____

Burial: _____

Do you want a listing on www.legacy.com or www.tributes.com (online guest book and messages of sympathy)?

_____

Is there any other information to be included in the obituary?

_____

_____

_____

If you can afford to print an obituary on two successive days, or if you want to print a shorter announcement on the second day, I encourage you to do so. Also, if the dying person was friends with their neighbors (or former neighbors), I recommend having a member of your family call one of the neighbors to tell her of your loved one's death and ask her to personally spread the word about memorial and funeral arrangements to the other neighbors (and former neighbors).

I assumed that at least one of my mother's neighbors would see my mother's obituary and inform the others. Unfortunately, none of her neighbors had read the newspaper on the only day that her obituary was printed, and so none the neighbors attended her memorial service. All expressed regret for having missed her burial and memorial services, and I expressed regret, too, at not having called one of them.

Be sure to ask a friend to go and purchase 5–20 of copies of the local newspaper (depending on your wishes) on the day that the obituary will run. You will want to have some originals to send to relatives and friends who live out of the area. It is also a good idea to create 10 or more photocopies of the obituary, since the original (on newsprint) will yellow over time, and you will also want to have photocopies to send to alumni magazines at high schools, colleges, and graduate schools; professional associations and/or unions, academic or religious fraternities, social clubs, a Council on Aging newsletter, and newsletters of civic or other groups to which your loved one has belonged.

Most alumni magazines or professional organizations will not publish news of someone's death unless a copy of a published obituary is submitted, with the name of the newspaper, city and state and date of publication written on it. If the obituary is not at the top of the page, so that the name of the newspaper and the date of publication is evident, then write the name of the newspaper, city, state and date of publication, as well as "Submitted by [YOUR NAME], address, and phone number," in the margin of the obituary before making copies of it. This will make it easier to send it to alumni associations, fraternal or union organizations, or other organizations that have newsletters or magazines in which you wish a death notice be printed.

Burial, Cremation, Funeral, Visiting Hours, and Memorial Service

Some people have very clear preferences about funeral arrangements, some do not have any preferences, and others do not want to think about such matters. Be sure to ask the dying person if he wants to be involved in planning his funeral arrangements.

Whether your loved one wishes to have you hold a simple memorial service or a multi-part wake/funeral/religious service/burial, many different types of memorial events can be arranged, involving special possessions of the person, special themes from the person's life, as well as involving many members of the family in different ways. For example, there can be many persons who walk alongside the casket, from children to elders, as honorary pallbearers, in addition to the persons who actually carry the casket.

If you decide to have speakers at a memorial or religious service, think carefully about who should speak. It is wise to limit their comments to a short amount of time, such as three or four minutes each and ask that they write out their comments and stick to the script. It is also helpful to advise speakers about what aspect of the loved one's life you wish them to address, so that you will not end up with the second and third speakers starting their comments with, "He stole my story, so I guess I will tell you about something else..."

If the dying person wishes to discuss funeral arrangements with you, you can use the form on pages 86–87 as a basis for discussion, or **you can order a sixteen page funeral planning kit "Before I Go You Should Know" from Funeral Consumers Alliance (see www.funerals.org),** which contains an explanatory booklet, forms to fill out, and a bright blue plastic folio in which to keep the information. The Funeral Consumers Alliance is a nonprofit organization that is dedicated to informing consumers about options for funeral and burial arrangements, including very low cost arrangements. If you like a "self-help" approach to educating yourself about subjects, I encourage you to visit the Funeral Consumers Alliance website, www.funerals.org to find out more about what these nonprofit, citizen led groups offer, and to read the articles that are available. While some funeral directors regard the Funeral Consumers Alliance as being "anti-funeral industry," and caution that their materials may not be accurate, the Funeral Consumers Alliance materials offer thought-provoking information that is worth reviewing.

The National Funeral Directors Association website, www.nfda.org, which represents licensed funeral home directors, is a resource for funeral directors as well as the public. At this site, you will find information concerning the role of funeral directors, the many types of services and products offered by funeral homes, and information concerning cremation and burial. For example, the site mentions the fact that pacemakers must be removed before cremation, for they could explode and cause injury or death to the crematory staff. This is an important consideration for families to be aware of. Also, the site explains that families who wish to have a viewing and then cremation may reduce their overall costs by paying a fee to use a rental casket for the viewing and then purchase an inexpensive container for the ashes.

As with any profession, there are ethical funeral directors who conduct their work from a place of deep service and there are other funeral directors who are in it primarily for the money. Looking at the professional side of the Funeral Home Directors Association site will give you a glimpse into the marketing focus of the funeral industry. This can help you prepare for any sales tactics that you may encounter.

There have been highly publicized cases in which prepaid funeral funds have gone missing, and others in which families' funds have been used to purchase high amounts of death benefit insurance on their loved ones (to benefit the funeral director above and beyond the services purchased), rather than the funds being placed directly in secure escrow accounts. In recent years there have also been several scandals concerning crematoriums and cemeteries. While such problems are statistically rare, it behooves all of us to be educated consumers about funeral home services, products and prepayment arrangements. Viewing both the Funeral Consumers Alliance website and the Funeral Directors Association website is a way to look at important issues concerning funerals from more than one viewpoint.

Religious Tradition and House of Worship

Be sure to ask the dying person if he wishes to follow traditions of a specific faith, and if there is a specific church, synagogue, mosque, or other location where he would want religious or other services held. Be sure to also ask if there is a specific clergyperson or lay member of a specific faith or tradition who should be consulted about the traditions to follow.

If your loved one believes in a religion but has not attended a house of worship for many years, nor been a paying member of a house of worship, but wants to have a memorial or religious service held in their memory, now is the time for you to contact their preferred house of worship and speak with the clergyperson concerning their policies and procedures regarding arrangements for services (both availability and cost). Many houses of worship schedule weddings and other celebrations up to a year in advance. Don't assume that you will be able to make one call to your preferred house of worship on the day that your loved one dies and be accommodated for a service a few days later.

Contacting the house of worship and clergyperson regarding their service arrangements can also be helpful in other ways. Often, religions have customs regarding cremation vs. burial, embalming or not embalming, whether to hold a wake with an open casket, type of casket, how soon the burial should occur, whether the family will invite their friends into their homes for prayers, etc. Since the dying person's preferences concerning their funeral plans may disregard some or all of these religious customs, you will want to check with the clergyperson to see if your loved one's decisions could have an impact on whether the funeral services, mass, or memorial service can be held in that religion's house of worship, and/or whether that specific clergyperson is willing to participate in a funeral or memorial service.

If you have discussed these matters with the dying person and you have their wishes recorded in writing (and signed by them, if possible), you will be able to use those writings as a basis for discussion with the clergyperson. Be sure to refer to that list as you ask the clergyperson if the dying person's specific wishes regarding funeral and memorial services can be accommodated, so that no details or specific wishes will be overlooked.

Pre-Arranging Funeral Services

Whether or not you know the wishes of the dying person concerning funeral and memorial service arrangements, I encourage you to investigate the range and cost of funeral services while your loved one is still living.

By pre-arranging or pre-planning, I do not mean to recommend pre-payment, unless you are in the process of qualifying for Medicaid, in which case pre-paying basic funeral costs makes financial sense. Basic funeral expenses are considered legitimate expenses that can be taken before all finances are paid down to the minimum $2,000 level that is allowed for Medicaid eligibility. If Medicaid eligibility is not a consideration, then please consider carefully the pros and cons of pre-payment of funeral expenses, including reading about prepayment scandals and how to avoid them, before making a financial commitment.

While making funeral arrangements in advance of someone's death is not an easy task, making such arrangements immediately following a death is even more difficult, in my personal experience. Therefore, I encourage you to learn about options for funeral arrangements and to consider how much you wish to do on your own, and how much you want the help of a funeral director.

I am very glad that I went to a funeral director to make my mother's funeral arrangements several months before she died. My siblings were not ready to consider my mother's funeral or memorial service arrangements, but they did not object to me doing so. Making the advance plans with the funeral director regarding the casket and flowers set in motion my ideas concerning her burial service and the memorial service. I then contacted a close friend of my mother's in her Bahá'í community and she and I designed the burial service and the memorial service and reception that would follow. Planning the burial and memorial services, as well as the post-memorial reception, with this friend and with other members of her Bahá'í community was a deeply moving process that allowed us to share stories of my mother that neither of us had known before. In this close collaboration, I was able to honor my mother's spirit and create a much more significant service than if I had had to do all of these preparations in the 24 hours after her passing.

Investigating funeral arrangements before the person actually dies is important in another respect: the cost of services provided by funeral homes varies widely. If you wait until a death to make such arrangements, you will not have the time to compare the value and cost of several different funeral service providers, and therefore you may end up paying thousands—if not tens of thousands—of dollars more than you need to for the same services that you could have had at another local funeral home. If you wish to learn about ways to limit expenditures for funeral arrangements, I encourage you to see the resources on the Funeral Consumers Alliance site www.funerals.org.

According to the 1984 Federal Trade Commission regulations, the general price list and a casket selection price list must be given to anyone asking for them, to enable families to see, up front, what the costs of different products and services will be. Unfortunately, in Massachusetts, the enforcement division has recently found that 30% or more of funeral homes are not complying with the law in this regard. A reputable funeral home will have nothing to hide and will be glad to honor your wishes to consider your options for services and costs, so do not settle for a verbal explanation of costs. It is your right to receive a copy of the general price list for funeral services, as well as a list of casket and burial vault options and costs, without having to make any commitment to use that funeral home.

If you are one of the many people, as I am, who subscribe to the "buy local" philosophy, you will want to inquire about whether the funeral home is independently owned and operated and whether it is a member of the *International Order of the Golden Rule* (www.ogr.org), an association of independently owned funeral homes that subscribe to ethical standards as well as commitments to be involved in their local communities. Locally owned funeral homes that are members of the *International Order of the Golden Rule* tend to use the services of local businesses, including banks, insurance agencies, florists and casket manufacturers, whereas funeral homes that are part of a national chain that may be headquartered thousands of miles away may or may not have a commitment to strengthening the local community by using local vendors.

One way to find out about the practices of funeral homes is to speak with families that have been helped by specific funeral homes. I also recommend that you visit several funeral homes before deciding to finalize a funeral plan, to see the layout of the rooms, to talk with the staff, and to see how much of the orientation of the funeral home is toward educating and helping the family, rather than simply selling products.

One funeral home that I visited, for example, had a wonderful lending library of books on topics related to death and dying, funerals, grief, and children and family issues. This lending library told me a great deal about the caring attitude of that funeral director. By making personal visits, you will be able to get a firsthand experience of how the funeral home director and staff relate to you, see the rooms in which visitation or memorial services would be held, hear about the services and philosophy of the funeral home, and be able to view the "merchandise" (the casket and burial vault). At each visit, be sure to ask for a price list detailing the general professional services cost, as well as costs of the casket, burial vault, limousines/ hearses, rental of rooms for services, and options such as embalming, cosmetics, hairdressing, and memorial cards or keepsakes, and take it home with you to review more thoroughly after the visit.

The casket and burial vault tend to be the most expensive parts of the funeral arrangements. Caskets can range from bio-degradable, cloth-covered paperboard or unstained wood boxes to elaborate wooden, metal (even precious metal), or stone caskets. Before deciding on choice of casket, I suggest checking with the cemetery to see if there is a requirement that the casket or urn be enclosed inside a vault for burial. If it is optional, you may choose to forego the expense of an outer burial vault. Note: By law, a funeral home cannot add charges if you wish to provide your own casket or burial vault. Although few people may wish to make their own arrangements for buying (or making) a casket or burial vault, there can be substantial savings to be had by doing so, and the Funeral Consumers Alliance (or online search engines) can provide information about casket and burial vault vendors.

If the body is to be buried within a few days, you will have the choice to embalm the body or not. Local ordinances may proscribe how long an unembalmed body can be kept before burial, but now most funeral homes have adequate facilities for holding a body, even one that is not embalmed, for several days to a week. Some religious traditions have preferences or dictates regarding embalming or not embalming. Consult the appropriate clergyperson for advice regarding embalming, if your loved one wishes to follow a specific religion's practices in this regard.

If your loved one wishes to be buried in a casket, you will want to think about whether you want to stay to see the casket lowered into the ground and have all of the dirt put over it. Many families do not stay for this final aspect of the burial, but some friends of mine said that they felt that they needed and wanted to be there as all of the dirt, not just a few symbolic handfuls, was used to fill up the grave.

If your loved one wishes to be cremated, you can ask if he has any preference regarding choice of urn (these can range from simple fiber containers to special hand-made urns of many different materials) and where he wishes to have his ashes interred, held, or scattered.

Specific wishes regarding burial (such as wanting the family to stay to see the grave filled in following the graveside ceremony) or cremation (where to have ashes interred or scattered), and selection of pallbearers (or honorary pallbearers who walk alongside the casket or urn but do not carry it) can be listed here:

_____

_____

_____

_____

Funeral Planning Check List

Funeral Home:_____

Funeral Home Director Name: _____Tel. _____

	Cost
Basic Services of Funeral Director and Staff	_____
Immediate Burial	_____
Direct Cremation	_____
Embalming	_____
Dressing/Casketing/Cosmetology/Haircare:	_____
Other Patient Care: _____	_____
Use of Facilities and Staff (viewing/visitation/wake)	_____
Use of Facilities and Staff (funeral ceremony)	_____
Use of Facilities and Staff (memorial service)	_____
Use of Facilities and Staff (graveside service)	_____
Use of Facilities and Staff (church/other service)	_____
Hearse for transfer	_____
Hearse for services	_____
Lead/clergy/flower car	_____
Limousines # _____Service Vehicle _____	_____
Casket Model: _____ Maker_____ Color_____	_____
Outer Burial Container Model _____	_____
Cremation Urn Model _____	_____
Memorial/Prayer Cards # _____	_____
Guest Register Book Type: _____	_____
Acknowledgment Cards:# _____	_____
DVD/Video- photos and music _____	_____
Other keepsakes: #____ Type _____	_____
Clothing (Maker/Style #)_____	_____
Death Certificates #____ Doctor:_____	_____

Burial/Disposition Permit:_____ _____

Obituary Newspaper1 (#days)_____ _____

Newspaper2 (#days)_____ _____

Cemetery:_____Sect:___Lot___Grave___ _____

Forwarding Remains to:_____ _____

Receiving Remains from:_____ _____

Other Fees/Services_____ _____

Total charges: _____

Cemetery Burials and Green Burials; Burying or Scattering Ashes

If the dying person wishes their body or ashes to be buried, do they already own a cemetery plot? If so, contact the cemetery to confirm the location of the plot and to confirm how much space is available in the plot. Single cemetery plots are designed to hold one casket, but can accommodate more than one cremation urn; double plots are designed to hold two caskets but can hold a number of cremation urns. Each cemetery will have its own regulations concerning how many urns are allowed, as well as whether an outside burial vault is required, and whether a "double plot" will allow two caskets to be buried side by side, or have the first casket buried deeper than usual, and the other buried on top of that one at a later date.

If the dying person wishes to have a burial, but does not own a cemetery plot, do they want to be buried in a particular cemetery, have their body or ashes interred in a mausoleum, or given a "green burial" in a peaceful, park-like setting that has been established for such purposes? Green burial cemeteries are a relatively new concept and they usually have different regulations from traditional cemeteries, such as forbidding headstones but allowing markers flush with the ground, to retain the natural landscape and avoid looking like a cemetery. To find out more about Green Burials, you can put Green Burials into an internet search engine, or check the Funeral Consumers Alliance site www.funerals.org.

It is also possible, at least in some locations, to be buried on private property that is not a cemetery, even in your own back yard. You would need to check with your local government or public health board regarding any regulations regarding burial on private land that is not designated as a cemetery.

There is an issue worth consideration regarding a burial on private land in a place other than a cemetery—the environmental impact of that action. Is the private land where a person wants to be buried appropriate for a burial? Is the water table high, or is there sufficient drainage? Is it part of a watershed connected to a drinking supply? These factors should be taken into consideration before making a decision that could have a negative environmental impact.

Even if it would be allowed to bury your loved one on your own property, and there are no environmental issues standing in the way of you doing so, you will want to consider whether this would present problems to selling the property in the future. Would you want to have to bring up this matter with future buyers of your home? I can envision a conversation going something like this, "Oh yes, one more thing—our Grandmother is buried next to the large oak in the back yard, and we want to have unfettered access to the burial site included in the deed of sale." That statement could make it impossible to sell a property, at any price.

Veterans' Benefits

If the person who is dying is a veteran who received a discharge (other than dishonorable), and you have his discharge papers (DD214) and a copy of his birth certificate (as well as marriage certificate, if you are seeking benefits for the surviving spouse), he will qualify for the following:

*Veteran grave marker. To find out more information about grave markers for veterans, call 1-800-697-6947 from 8 am until 5 pm, Monday through Friday, except federal holidays, or consult the website www.cem.va.gov.

*American flag at the funeral service.

If the veteran meets certain eligibility conditions, the veteran may also qualify for:

*Basic burial allowance of $300.

*Plot or interment allowance of $150.

*Burial in a veterans' cemetery.

For complete information regarding veterans death benefits, call your local veterans office, or go to the website www.va.gov or call 1-800-827-1000.

A funeral director will usually assist you in filling out the forms for Veterans Benefits.

Notes/questions regarding veteran benefits:

_____

_____

_____

Headstone

If the person wishes to be buried in a cemetery, consult with the cemetery administrator concerning the type and size of headstones that are allowed. Then, ask the dying person what type of headstone she wishes to have (color, type and shape of stone or other material). What name (first or nickname, middle, last, suffix) does she want on the stone? What other wording does she wish to have written on the head stone? Are there religious or other symbols that he wishes to have etched into the stone? If the person has died before you select a headstone, I suggest that you confirm the full spelling of your loved one's first, middle and last names (and any suffix, if used), as well as his birth date, via his birth certificate or other legal document in advance of ordering the stone. This is not the time to rely on your memory, or even what you have been told by other family members, because **errors are very costly to correct on an engraved headstone.**

As with making funeral arrangements in advance of a death, I encourage you to take the time to compare vendors for headstones in advance of the death of your loved one. You will be surprised at the different stone types and design options that vendors offer, and also by the great difference in costs for identical headstones or markers. Talking to several vendors, when you are not rushed to make a decision, can save you thousands of dollars as well as giving you more time to make such important decisions as the shape, size, color, design elements and wording of the headstone or marker.

Social Security Benefits

There is a small "lump sum" benefit that is available to the surviving widow or widower (at the time of this writing it is $255). Usually, the funeral director will forward a statement of death (Funeral Home Director Form SSA-721) to your Social Security Office. *It is the responsibility of the surviving spouse or guardian of dependent children to contact the Social Security Office within seven days of the death, to prevent possible loss of benefits. Please visit the website* www.socialsecurity.gov *or call 1-800-772-1213 from 7am-7pm, Monday through Friday.*

Personalizing Memorial Services

It is worth remembering that the wake (also known as visiting hours or calling hours) and the memorial service are not for your deceased loved one, nor are they only for you, but they are for the friends and family members who will feel the need to say good-bye and honor him. Even the keepsakes (prayer cards or other mementos) can be very important to the people who come to pay their respects. *One friend told me that his 94 year old godmother said, "When I want to visit my friends, I go through the prayer cards and think of them and remember the good times that we had together."* For this person, a prayer card from a wake is a tangible symbol of a person and their life, to be treasured and remembered on an ongoing basis.

When one of our elderly family members died, a person of my generation said, "Why hold a memorial service? All of her friends are dead." This ended up not being the case—about 80 family members and friends attended the memorial service for that elderly person. This taught me an important lesson—no matter how old a deceased person is, there will probably be individuals who need to attend the service to pay their respects and say good-bye. A memorial service creates a sacred space into which all who feel moved to attend the ceremony can do so.

Of course, if you feel strongly that you cannot cope with the stress of arranging a memorial service, or your loved one wished that services be private, or there is another overriding reason to not hold any services, then not holding services may be the best option.

Perhaps the religious tradition of your loved one will dictate the elements of funeral services and the order in which they occur, but if you are not bound by religious customs, it is worth considering which elements of such services are ones that you wish to have, and in which order.

A traditional sequence for funeral services is usually to have a wake (visiting hours, with an open or closed casket or a cremation urn), then a funeral (a final meeting of relatives and friends at the funeral home, with brief prayers or readings, followed by a funeral procession), then a funeral Mass or church or synagogue service, and then the burial in a cemetery (the burial can be private, or open to the public). However, many of the funeral home sites that I visited on the internet emphasized the endless variety of services as well as sequences of elements that are possible, and a willingness to have the family design each part of the funeral arrangements in a way that honors the deceased person's religious or cultural values, wishes, and interests.

In the case of my mother's services, we held her burial in the mid-morning, we held a Bahá'í memorial service in a private home immediately following the burial, then we offered a luncheon reception in the same home. This sequence of ceremonies allowed family and friends to say goodbye to her physical form and then celebrate her life. A couple who attended my mother's memorial service, who were also caring for their elderly mother, commented on how wonderful it was to end on a happy note rather than with the burial service, and they decided to hold their mother's burial before the church memorial service when their own mother died about six months later.

Reception

It is entirely up to you as to whether you hold a reception after a funeral service, religious service, or memorial service. Some families designate a local restaurant at which families and friends are invited to gather for food and drinks. Choosing to hold a meal or reception at a restaurant is the most expensive option, especially if you provide alcoholic beverages, but it does have clear advantages: you get to determine how long the gathering lasts, and the staff does the set-up and clean-up. In fact, if you are tired, you can leave the reception when you desire and leave your guests to continue without you.

If you wish to further reduce the cost of a reception, you can explore whether or not the house of worship in which the memorial service will be held is able to hold a reception in another part of the building or if there is a space nearby that can be rented. In these cases, you might have an option of hiring a caterer, or in some cases, a women's service group connected with the house of worship can provide some or all of the refreshments, either for low cost or no cost (this usually depends on how involved with the congregation the deceased individual or their family has been).

Many times, families do not hold any public reception, but instead invite only the closest relatives and friends to share a meal or light refreshments at a club, restaurant, or private home. If the loved one has been cared for in your home, I suggest using another location for this gathering. Chances are, you have been too exhausted to keep up with housekeeping, and the last thing you should concern yourself with now is doing a thorough cleaning of your home in order to receive guests.

If your loved one has not given you clear instructions regarding a reception, it may help to think of what your loved one would have wanted you to do.

My parents, teenagers during the Great Depression, would have been horrified if we had spent a lot of money paying for food at a restaurant, since they almost never "ate out" due to their strong feelings that it was a waste of money to do so. Having a private reception in our home following my father's death, and a reception in the home of one of my mother's Bahá'í friends following my mother's burial, was a way of honoring each of their values while creating a much more intimate setting for sharing stories about their lives.

CHAPTER SEVEN

HOSPICE CARE

- Definition of Hospice
- When to Seek Hospice Care
- 24 Hour a Day, On-call Support
- Where Hospice Care Can Be Delivered

Definition of Hospice

Hospice care has been a wonderful program for my dying relatives and friends, and I deeply believe in its philosophy and benefits. Since it is so poorly understood in the United States, I hope to clarify its purpose for those who have not yet seen the benefits of hospice care for a dying person. (For more information about the hospice movement, please see the websites listed on page 162.)

Briefly stated, the purpose of hospice care is to provide "comfort care" to those who have been diagnosed with a condition that is terminal, that is, when a cure is not possible and the person is likely to live six months or less. "Comfort care" means that the emphasis of the care is changed from finding a cure to providing the most comfortable, supportive, respectful, and pain-free environment in which people can live out their natural lives, as the medical condition progresses toward death. This "comfort care" approach emphasizes pain relief and symptom relief and places the welfare and wishes of the patient as the most important areas of focus in caregiving.

It also integrates counseling, group support, and spiritual support, as requested by the family. This multi-dimensional approach creates an environment that honors the patient's and family's desires for privacy, peace, and connection. It is in stark contrast to the Western medical model, in which increasing amounts of pharmaceuticals and medical interventions are utilized to extend the life of the person, regardless of the quality of his life or the amount of pain to which he is subjected.

In the traditional medical model, death represents failure on the part of the doctors and the medical system. Within this model, chronic and acute pain are often under-treated out of a fear that the person will become addicted to pain medication or they will die sooner due to the pain medication. Very little time is spent by many

93

physicians discussing the pluses and minuses of any given medical treatment, the likelihood of complications and adverse outcomes of these treatment options, or alternative options for treatment. The unfortunate consequence of how the traditional medical system operates is that many times, elderly persons are subjected to medical tests and treatments that are painful in themselves and may only extend their lives for days or weeks, with little quality of life and continual pain.

When I worked as a housekeeper in an assisted living facility, I knew an elderly resident who had intense back pain due to calcification of her spine. She chose to undergo a very invasive surgical procedure, removing the calcium deposits from the length of her spinal column, with the promise that it would allow her freedom from pain and greater mobility. According to the doctors, the operation was a success—they removed the calcium deposits and there were no infections after the surgery—but the operation failed totally in giving her relief from pain or increasing her mobility. She died a few months after the surgery, after having endured constant pain that was worse than the pain before the surgery and all the while being completely bedridden. The pain medication that was given to her was given infrequently, in spite of her intense suffering. I remembered thinking, "There must be a better way to help dying people than this."

Hospice care is designed to provide your loved one with the highest quality of life during whatever time she has left to live. The social workers, nurses, CNAs, chaplains and physicians who are hospice providers have a deep understanding of the many aspects of the dying process—physical, mental, and spiritual. This cross-disciplinary understanding is often missing in the training and experience of regular physicians and nurses. Even if the physician is particularly knowledgeable about such matters, the insurance industry does not reimburse physicians for the time spent discussing treatment options and end of life care options, so little time is allotted for these discussions in most cases.

When to Seek Hospice Care

Hospice care does not require a diagnosis of cancer or of any specific disease. Persons of any age may be admitted to hospice care when they no longer seek a cure and when a doctor determines they will probably not live more than six months.

Since hospice care is for persons for whom a "cure" is no longer possible, hospices may require that the person who is admitted to hospice care forego medical interventions and procedures such as surgery, chemotherapy, radiation, and pharmaceuticals that are designed to cure an illness. Hospice care can permit "maintenance" medications (ones that treat underlying, long term conditions) and medications that alleviate pain or physical symptoms such as nausea, vertigo, constipation or diarrhea, or psychological conditions such as depression or anxiety. It is this in-depth knowledge with end of life care that hospice physicians and nurses bring to their work that can dramatically improve the quality of life for a dying person.

Hospice care greatly benefited my father, who was dying of both lung and heart disease. As he neared the end of his life, he was struggling for breath even while connected to an oxygen tank on the highest level of oxygen. He developed such a fear of not being able to breathe while lying down that he stayed sitting up in his lounge chair all night instead of going to bed. This did not allow him the replenishment of deep sleep, and he became exhausted and irritable.

As part of his admission to hospice care, the social worker and medical team of hospice did a thorough physical and mental assessment of my father, and correctly determined that my father's anxiety was worsening his ability to breath. Once they prescribed an appropriate anti-anxiety medication for him, he was able to breath more freely and no longer feared going to bed. Once he was able to sleep in his bed at night, he became relaxed, his old personality returned, and he was able to enjoy his last days of living. His comment to me, said in a jaunty voice, was "If this is dying, dying ain't bad!" Having seen the dramatic improvement that hospice had made in his life, I wished we had convinced his doctor to evaluate him for hospice care at a much earlier time, or that we had approached hospice directly for an evaluation.

If the patient's physician is not supportive of referring the patient to hospice care, I encourage you to contact the local hospice intake coordinator directly, to speak about the patient's condition and to discuss the possibility of having a different doctor evaluate the dying person. Once the patient has been referred to hospice, the hospice team can meet with the family to discuss the appropriateness of hospice care and evaluate the needs of the dying person.

24 Hour-a-Day On-Call Support

The hospice care team, consisting of a hospice physician, nurse, social worker, and spiritual counselor or chaplain (if requested), will assist you in creating a plan of care that works for you and your loved one. They are available 24 hours a day via phone, should you have questions and concerns, and a hospice nurse can be dispatched to the site, if necessary. Knowing this will be an immense comfort to you, whether you are caring for your loved one at home or in another setting.

Where Hospice Care Can Be Delivered

Hospice care can be delivered to a person in her home, at a live-in hospice, or in another setting, such as a nursing home. If the patient is in a nursing home or other facility, once the patient has been admitted to hospice care, the hospice team will take over the management of all medications. This is a very important transfer of power, for often traditional medical staff are not trained in the appropriate use of pain medication and other comfort care at the end of life.

A cautionary note is needed here: *I have been disappointed to realize, through personal experience, that some nursing home staff will give inaccurate information to the hospice staff in an effort to circumvent hospice care. If your loved one continues to be in pain even hours after pain-relieving medication has been prescribed by the hospice physician, I encourage you to notify the hospice team directly so that they can assess the situation and take immediate action to relieve the suffering of your loved one.*

Note: If your loved one is under the care of hospice at the time of his or her death, the hospice nurse will not only come to check the person's vital signs and pronounce the person dead, but she will also immediately remove any prescriptive pain medicines that the hospice had provided. It is important to know that this isn't a sign of someone "being too business-like," but rather this protocol must be followed to ensure that pain medicines will not be abused by others or sold on the black market.

CHAPTER EIGHT

WHERE TO CARE FOR YOUR LOVED ONE

- Staying at Home
- At Home Equipment Needs
- Continuum of Care Facilities
- Independent Living
- Assisted Living
- Skilled Nursing
- If a Nursing Home Is the Only or Best Choice
- Quality at the End of Life Depends on Time Spent with Your Loved One
- Form Relationships with Nursing Home Staff
- Form a Self-Help Support Network of Family Caregivers
- Change Comes, Though Slowly

The decision about whether to have your loved one stay at home, move in with someone else, or move to an assisted living/ nursing facility, or hospice is at the heart of "caring well." Choosing the most appropriate setting in which to die will determine the extent to which the dying person is able to maintain a level of individual control over the most intimate details of his life, as well as providing a comfortable environment in which to live out his final months, days, and hours.

What is the "best" environment for the dying person? Referring to your answers in the survey in Chapter Four will help you to understand what factors contribute to your loved one's quality of life. For some persons, the prospect of moving to a nursing facility may offer benefits such as companionship, planned activities, and ready-made meals.

Others, particularly persons who are shy or introverted, may feel that being around many people in a structured environment would be very distasteful to them. They would rather live in their current home or apartment, with all of their possessions around them and with a sense of privacy. For those persons, a move to an institutional setting with different structures and rigid schedules can be a traumatic experience, leading to profound depression. (I encourage you to read the book "*Senior Power*," listed on page 158, by the late Dr. Clifford Bennett, a nursing home administrator who signed himself into an out-of-state nursing home as part of his doctoral dissertation and reported on life inside a nursing home from a resident's perspective. It is a powerful recounting of the psychological changes that he experienced as a nursing home resident, even though he knew what nursing homes were like from an administrator's point of view.)

I have interviewed many people concerning their wishes for end of life care. I have yet to meet someone who hopes that they will die in a nursing home, and I have yet to meet a resident of a nursing home who would not want to leave the nursing home, if at home care were an option. This is not to say that nursing homes are not needed for end of life care. Many people will end up living their last days in a nursing home because at home care is not available, for any number of reasons.

My personal experiences in caring for loved ones in nursing home settings have led me to *the conclusion that the nursing home industry as it currently exists is a broken system*. Nursing homes, except for some entirely "private pay" facilities and the unusual homes that have substantial endowments, are terribly underfunded by insurance, Medicare and Medicaid, resulting in inadequate, impersonal care for large numbers of senior citizens and underpaid (and non-benefitted) caregivers, especially certified nursing assistants (CNAs). These CNAs, who do the labor intensive, hands on care of toileting, bathing and feeding residents, are often not provided with health insurance, sick days, vacation days, or paid holidays. Consequently, morale is low and turnover is high. This, in turn, makes facilities rely heavily on "pool" or "agency" (temporary) certified nursing assistants, who do not know the residents and often do not even read care plans.

Unfortunately, many people who choose to enter the attractive doors of "continuing care" communities as residents of independent living or assisted living units, and who enjoy their time in those environments, are completely unaware of the lack of independence, loss of personal control, and inadequate staffing (especially from 7 pm until 7 am) that they will experience living in the nursing home during the final stage in their journey.

Staying at Home

Remaining at home to die, whether in their own home or in yours, offers many advantages to a dying person. Perhaps the most obvious, but often undervalued, is the comfort of staying in their known surroundings, with the furnishings, objects, scenery, sounds (or quiet), and smells that they know and love.

Many elderly persons have some degree of dementia, and staying at home, or in a known environment (such as the home of a relative) enables them to cope to the best of their abilities. In contrast, moving them from the environment that they knew and loved to an entirely new environment such as a nursing home causes the symptoms of their dementia to become more acute.

Most important, the decision to live and die at home will usually allow the dying person a greater amount of individual control over her most personal decisions: when to sleep, when to be alone or with others, when (and what) to eat, and when to use the toilet, versus having these activities be dictated by an institution's schedule, protocols, and staffing levels. The exception to this generalization is live-in hospices, which strive to give full control to each resident concerning their sleep schedule, as well as eating, toileting, and other activities.

The most frequent concerns that result in not keeping a chronically ill or dying person at home are the cost of at home care, fear for the dying person's safety, and personal fear of not being able to render 24-hour a day care that someone would get in a nursing facility.

It is important to note that not all persons with terminal diagnoses will require 24-hour a day care until some time further along in their illness. If they do not, you might wish to explore the idea of utilizing an "Adult Day Care" in your area (see page 157), if your loved one needs assistance, medication, and activities during the day but you are able to provide care in the evening and overnight. If you need paid helpers, there are many sources for at home caregivers, including Councils on Aging, visiting nurses associations, hospices, and independent health care agencies (see pages

157, 162, 163, 165). I encourage you to explore at home care options thoroughly before deciding to choose a nursing home care option, as home care can provide a much higher quality of care.

The cost associated with staying at home is dependent on several factors: the degree to which the dying person is able and willing to be alone for periods of time versus their need or wish for companionship and assistance; the degree to which he or she can or cannot do (or help with) any basic activities of daily life such as eating, using the bathroom, and taking medications; the availability or lack of availability of family and friends to volunteer their time as caretakers; the simplicity or complexity of medical care that is needed and wanted by the dying person, and the type and degree of dementia that the dying person has. If your loved one has dementia, it is important to connect with The Alzheimer's Association (www.alz.org, page 158) to become knowledgeable about the progression of the disease.

It is not easy to care for a relative at your home or add overnight shifts of caregiving at their home to an already full life. In each of the situations in which I have cared for relatives or loved ones in their own homes, we have made some kind of space where an overnight caregiving relative or friend could stay and get some rest, if not full sleep, while taking an overnight shift. Having a fold-out day bed, couch, or even a camping mattress on the floor, will make the overnight responsibilities much more manageable for family volunteers. In the last few years, "baby monitors" have become quite advanced in their technology. Using them, it may be possible to lie down in another room yet be able to respond if your loved one speaks, responds, makes noise, or asks for help.

Spending time with a loved one in their final months, weeks and days in their own home also makes possible being with them in some remarkable moments in a way that would not be possible if they were in a nursing home setting. For example, people who are very elderly or dying often become more active after sun down, and then they want to sleep all day. Therefore, being with a loved one in the late evening and overnight may allow you to be with her when she is more active or alert versus seeing her when she is sleeping all day.

At Home Equipment Needs

If you care for your loved one in his home, you will want to arrange to rent equipment that can make your caregiving more manageable. I encourage you to do so before you actually need it, because you will never be able to predict when you will need it!

At 7 pm on a Saturday night, my father suddenly lost his ability to walk, even with a walker. Yet, his mind was still alert, and he insisted on using the bathroom. There was no service agency available at that hour from which we might rent a wheelchair. We were lucky that a member of our family worked in a medical setting and had access to borrow a folding wheelchair until Monday morning, but if this hadn't been the case, we would not have had a solution to our problem.

The medical equipment that you will need includes:

- Hospital bed and pressure-relieving bed cushion
- Soaker pads (plastic-lined absorbent (disposable or reusable) pads to place under the person), which can also be used to move the person in their bed
- Walker
- Folding wheelchair
- Bedside commode with arms
- Bedpan
- High seat and arms to go over the toilet, so that the person can more safely and easily use the toilet
- A transfer bench for the bathtub or shower, to enable someone to sit down and then slide over, as needed

In addition, you will want to purchase the following:

- Disposable briefs (Depends or other brands). If your loved one is able to help with changing these, pull-on ones are best. Otherwise, choose ones with tabs that can be put on and taken off more easily, even if someone is unconscious or unable to help in the process.

- Vinyl disposable gloves. Buy a box of 100, rather than a small package, to save on the cost.

- Box of face masks to prevent coughing or sneezing in the ill person's presence. Note: a tiny amount of natural room freshener can be put onto the face mask of the provider to help mask odors, if desired.

- Baby wipes. Some have aloe and vitamin E and are more gentle on the skin.

- Paper towels. Get a big package of 10 rolls or so.

- Extra bath and hand towels, washcloths, sheets, and pillow cases.

- Extra garbage bags.

- Bendable beverage straws or a child's closed "sippy cup," to assist someone in drinking while in bed.

- A blender, if someone needs to eat pureed food.

- Bottles or cans of Ensure or another such nutritional beverage, to give someone nutrition even if they cannot eat food.

- Extra laundry detergent, surface cleaner, and other cleaning supplies.

- A can of natural, non-aerosol room freshener (I prefer a natural citrus scent available in health food stores). Once you begin to care for someone's bodily needs, it is helpful to be able to eliminate odors that are unpleasant from their living space, and for your own sake.

Continuum of Care Facilities

Many facilities that care for the elderly now advertise themselves as offering continuing care, in other words, independent living, assisted living, and skilled nursing care, all within the same community. This continuum of care concept is theoretically a good model, so that elders will not be required to leave the facility and find a new one as their needs for medical and personal care increase.

I know firsthand that many independent living and assisted living facilities are wonderful. They are lovely, happy places where residents have their privacy, retain control over many aspects of their lives, and enjoy nice surroundings and companionship.

However, the last stage of the continuum of care—the skilled nursing facility—is almost always sorely lacking in privacy, control, and enjoyment. Before you encourage your loved one to move to an independent living or assisted living facility, be sure to visit the skilled nursing facility (or dementia unit) several times, not only in the daytime but also in the evening from 8-9:30 pm, to become realistic in your expectations of what life there will be like. Once your loved one has been admitted to either an independent or assisted living facility, there is a likelihood that the progression of their disease will mean that they will eventually reside in the nursing care or dementia unit.

It is critical to realize that from the time of admission to an independent living or assisted living facility, control of what happens next is largely taken out of your hands. Your loved one is only one accident or one fall away from being declared by the nursing staff or administrators as inappropriate for the level of care at which he was admitted, and he will be required to move to the next level of care.

Independent Living

Independent living is a term used for several types of community housing, usually for persons 55 years of age or older. Independent living units may be apartments within a building, townhouse (condo-type) homes, or separate houses within an independent living community. The health criteria for entering an independent living unit vary from organization to organization, but usually require that the person be ambulatory or able to get from place to place via a wheelchair or with a walker; be mentally alert and able to live alone; be able to take their own medications, and provide most of their own personal care, with some assistance by a CNA.

Many independent living communities provide amenities such as beautiful architecture and landscaping, concierge services, and restaurant quality dining rooms. Some require upfront purchase of the villa, condo, or apartment, in addition to the payment of monthly residence fees; other facilities allow rental of the unit, in addition to the monthly residence fee.

Again, I offer a word of warning if you encourage your loved one to become a resident of a wonderful independent living facility— unless you thoroughly investigate the nursing home unit before making this decision, you may be disappointed to find that the level of nursing home care is dramatically inferior to what they will experience in the independent living unit.

If you do decide that an independent living unit is the right place for your loved one to live, be sure to read the fine print on every page of the contract. This is not the time to give the contract a cursory look. There can be many hidden fees contained in the document, as well as clauses that may not guarantee the availability of care on the next level.

Assisted Living

The admission criteria for assisted living units usually preclude the admission of a dying person. Persons in assisted living must be ambulatory or able to transport themselves to a dining area via their own wheelchairs; must be able to take their own medication and feed themselves; and be able to dress/undress and toilet themselves with very little assistance (up to one hour per day of assistance is usually provided by a certified nursing assistant to each resident).

In my experiences visiting relatives or friends in assisted living environments, I have found them to be very nice places to live. If your loved one is currently ambulatory and able to care for him/her self in most regards, she may greatly enjoy living in an assisted living community. However, it is an important consideration to note that a change in the health status (for example, a stroke, a fall, or for any reason becoming unable to do daily living tasks) can be the basis for immediately disqualifying someone to stay on that assisted living unit.

My mother was not happy when we moved her from her home to the assisted living unit of a continuum of care facility, but she quickly adapted to living in her private room (into which we had moved several pieces of her furniture and photographs and knickknacks) and enjoyed the privacy of its private bathroom. She was fortunate enough to have a lovely resident from across the hall befriend her. This resident brought her to every activity and would go for walks with her. Everything was contained within a short distance and under one roof—the dining room, the hairdresser, and the activity room. Life seemed to be going splendidly for my mother, when only six weeks into her stay, she had another stroke that put her in a bed-ridden state for several days. This is when the fine print of the contract kicked in. As someone not able to care for herself, my mother now needed individualized care, 24 hours a day, seven days a week. We hired outside certified nursing assistants to provide that care at $22 per hour for several days. We were then advised that our mother was no longer appropriate for the assisted living unit and that she would have to move to the nursing unit. This is how the system moves individuals along according to its rules and regulations.

Skilled Nursing

Let me address three very important problems that are inherent in any nursing homes, *including skilled nursing facilities and skilled nursing wings in communities that market themselves as "continuing care" (or continuum of care) communities,* since many residents who love their independent living and assisted living quarters will eventually be moved to skilled nursing (or skilled nursing dementia) units. These problems are:

- Loss of personal control by the patient and family in virtually all aspects of the dying person's life
- Inadequate staff response times and errors, due to understaffing and staffing by per diem and "agency" temporary staff
- Lack of infection control and monitoring of safety of patients
- Patients' loss of physical strength and increase in psychological problems

I cannot emphasize enough that the move to a nursing level facility was experienced as a profound loss by all of the residents I came to know well while caring for my mother in the nursing home. Every person stated that they would give anything to be able to leave the nursing home and go back to their own home to die. Unfortunately, most families who make the decision to move their loved one to a nursing home are usually unwilling to consider alternative arrangements, once they have made this choice. This may be true because of the sale of the home or relinquishment of their apartment. Or it may simply be that the family is unwilling to consider other arrangements once their loved one has three meals a day and is receiving what they believe to be "excellent care."

No matter how elegant a nursing home looks, and many are elegantly furnished with antiques, art, curios in cabinets, chandeliers or grand pianos, the sad fact is that almost every nursing care facility in the United States is understaffed, especially on the evening and overnight shifts This inevitably results in institutionalized care regimens that ignore residents' wishes and desires and which contribute to the loss of vitality and strength on the part of residents. (In spite of the fact that the "Bill of Rights" posted on the wall may guarantee that the resident's wishes will be honored.)

When you go to visit a nursing home for the first time, a very "perky" marketing person will give you a guided tour of the establishment. This tour will always be arranged during the day, to coincide with maximum nursing, maintenance, and administrative staffing levels, as well as to show off special programs that are offered during daytime hours. This tour is designed to show the institution in the best possible light. He or she will probably introduce you to the most cogent and verbal residents, you will be shown a resident's room that is nicely outfitted, and staff will take the time to speak with you and show an interest in you and your loved one.

Although the person showing you around will not be called a salesperson, make no mistake about it—this is the *sales department* at work! It is the job of the staff member who will give you a tour of the facility to sell you on the benefits of deciding to move your loved one to their facility.

It is your job, as your dying relative or friend's caregiver, to get below the surface appearances to understand both the pluses and minuses of the particular establishment. To do so will require some research on your part, as well as a willingness to visit that facility un-announced on more than one occasion, especially *during the evening shift between the hours of 8:00-9:30 pm*. This will allow you to see what percentage of residents have been put to bed by 8:30 or 9:00 or 9:30 pm, and to hear how many "call bells" are sounding (and/or how many lights are lit outside of someone's door, indicating a request for help), which is an important indicator of whether or not the facility is adequately staffed.

Sometimes, nursing facilities will have signs saying "Preferred visiting hours are 11:00 am-8:00 pm." If the nursing home does not encourage visitors after 8:00 pm, this is one sign of understaffing on the evening shift. However, allowing visitors in the evening is no guarantee of adequate, quality care, since so few relatives or friends of residents ever come in the evening hours. Nursing home administrators count on the fact that the families of residents *almost never visit their loved ones after 6:00 pm*, and they will not expect you to do so, either.

When you take the official tour, be sure to bring a small pad and pen with you, to take down the names and titles of staff with whom you speak (and names of residents, and anything you want to remember about them, too). This will allow you to come back another day from 8:00-9:30 pm, to meet the nurses and staff in the evening, to talk with the same residents again, and simply to observe how smoothly the facility operates in the evening. This is the time you will find out how things *really* are in the lives of the residents! For example, you may find that there are many residents sitting in wheelchairs in a lounge, with no activity or music playing, and no staff members to keep them company. You will also be able to observe how many "call bells" (requests for assistance from the residents) and personal alarms are sounding (when residents on pressure sensitive alarm pads set off their alarms when they stand up) and what the response time is to those calls for help. You will also be able to hear how many residents are complaining about not being put to bed at their preferred bedtime, which is one of the chronic problems in nursing homes.

Nursing homes and skilled nursing facilities must meet minimum state certification standards for such facilities, but these minimal standards are woefully inadequate. State regulations regarding nursing home care, and Medicaid reimbursement for nursing care services, are constructed to be so minimal that the quality and amount of personal care available to each resident is barely adequate, at best, and shamefully inadequate in many instances.

The minimum square footage required in nursing home rooms in the state of Massachusetts is barely large enough to accommodate a hospital bed, one small chair, and a nightstand for each resident. Given the fact that closets, doors, windows, and built in bureaus can take up most of the perimeter of a resident's room, and there are fixed "privacy curtain tracks" in the ceiling of most rooms, there is little flexibility in the placement of furniture. The small amount of space allotted to each resident in many nursing homes precludes the elder from having the option of bringing in many pieces of his furniture, or of having many personal possessions. It also makes it nearly impossible to have peace and quiet if the other resident decides to keep the television turned on at a high volume.

It is usually the case that two residents will share a room, with only privacy curtains separating the living spaces. If you take a moment to think about it, most people who are admitted to nursing homes have not shared a room with anyone but their spouse for the last 50 or more years, and some have not shared a room with anyone since they were children. It is entirely unnatural to expect someone who has enjoyed her privacy for half a century or more to be put into a room with a complete stranger (sometimes more than one stranger) and expect her to feel "at home" in that situation.

Often, two adjoining rooms with two persons in each room must share one small bathroom that is built between the two rooms, even if two men live in one room and two women live in the other room. This can be very problematic and even dangerous for elders, many of whom have urinary or bowel urgency problems (needing to use the toilet frequently) combined with dementia (an inability to remember to knock on the door before entering the toilet room).

If you are considering putting your relative in a nursing home, I suggest that you visit www.medicare.gov/nhcompare to read the ratings for the facilities that you are considering. Ratings can help you to research the quality of care, as evaluated by an impartial, outside review team, and to review the team's specific findings. The Medicare government website will also spell out state regulations for such facilities, such as how many licensed practical or registered nurses must be available on each shift, the minimum requirements for patient-staff ratios, and procedures for reporting elder abuse or filing grievances with nursing homes.

Loss of Control on the Part of Residents and Inadequate Staff Response Times

Even the best nursing homes have been forced, through inadequate Medicare and Medicaid reimbursements, to streamline their operations to such a degree that personalized attention and care are sorely lacking. It is not unusual to have residents wait a half-hour, forty minutes, or even longer for someone to answer their call bell for toilet assistance in the evening hours. This can lead to great discomfort on the part of residents, to the point of emotional frustration and physical agony.

Since many elderly residents prefer to go to bed between 7 and 8 pm, and almost all residents in nursing homes require one-on-one assistance (and some require two assistants) to use the toilet and prepare for going to bed, it is impossible to fulfill all residents' desires in a timely way.

It is not unusual for residents to be put to bed an hour, two hours, or even three hours later than they want to go to bed. In some nursing homes, in an attempt to please some of the people some of the time, a resident may be put to bed at 7:00 pm one night, and at 9:30 or 10:00 pm the next.

The same inconsistency of assistance happens on the early morning shift, when a resident can be awakened at 5:30 am one morning and at 7:30 or 8:00 am the next morning. These wildly fluctuating schedules of bedtime care and morning care—with no coordination of the two—can result in ongoing sleep deprivation due to disruption of the residents' sleep cycles.

Ask yourself this—how well would you function, and feel, if you were forced to comply with bedtimes and wake-up calls that varied by as much as three or four hours on a day-to-day basis, and over which you had no control? It would be like having a three to four hour jet lag every few days!

Nursing home administrators will invariably deny huge discrepancies in morning and nighttime routines, or inordinately long response times, because they know fully well that very few (if any) of the residents are physically or mentally capable of remembering or taking notes about the long response time for a toilet request or a request to be put to bed that is ignored.

On the nursing home hall on which my mother lived, only one resident was cognitively strong enough to able to recount in detail the frustrations she had felt in the last day due to unanswered call bells or rude treatment by staff members. The rest of the residents were suffering from either dementia or physical conditions that rendered them unable to recount the frustrating incidents that were taking place and their feelings at the time of those events.

The only way that you will know the degree of responsiveness of the staff is if you go in the evening hours and take actual notes regarding when a resident's call light goes on and when the staff member actually arrives to give care; in many instances, staff arrive immediately simply to reset the call button and tell Jane Doe, "I will be with you in two or three minutes," although they then disappear for another twenty or more minutes. This disingenuous action can allow the staff to record fast response times in their care log, although actual care is not delivered at the time that the call button is reset. Although a resident may not be able to read a clock or write notes about when they requested help, this does not diminish residents' frustrations at having to wait for a long time after their bladder is telling them to urinate or their body is aching to be put in bed.

Nutrition and Hydration

Inadequate staffing and budget constraints take their toll on residents in other ways, as well. I have already discussed the disruptions and frustrations that persons living in nursing homes experience with regard to their wishes regarding sleeping and use of the toilet. The final frustration many nursing home residents experience is regarding the food they are served and the setting in which it is served.

While the printed menus seemed to offer adequate choices, the reality of the dining hall experience in the nursing home in which my mother lived did not match the menu or the marketing pitch. Sometimes the food listed on the public menu was not the same food that was being served. Oftentimes, the dining hall was out of residents' favorite foods, such as vanilla and chocolate ice cream, but instead had only "designer" flavors, such as "strawberry cheesecake" and "apple pie." Seeing the displeasure of the residents at being told that the only ice cream available was two flavors they didn't like, I could not understand why a dining service would allow itself to run out of vanilla and chocolate ice cream on a regular basis, yet purchase odd flavors that no one wanted but which then had to be served until used up.

I have also seen firsthand, on many occasions, forty or fifty nursing home residents sitting in a silent dining room for half an hour, waiting for their food to be served by only one or two servers. This understaffing also meant that staff didn't even take the time to inform the resident of menu choices, but would simply bring a selection to the resident whether he wanted it or not. Or, if the resident said he did not want the entrée selections, the staff would neglect to mention to the resident that he could choose any of several sandwich choices as an alternate meal, but would only offer a peanut butter and jelly sandwich.

I also observed on numerous occasions that residents who asked to be served coffee or tea would have to ask several times, or would finally give up in quiet resignation when the staff never followed through with the promised beverage. The sense of frustration on the part of the residents in the dining hall was almost always evident. When I brought my observations and concerns to the dining room manager, his response was firm and non-empathic, "The budget doesn't allow me to hire more staff."

When my mother's energy and appetite declined following an illness, we requested that a small bowl of fruited yogurt (any brand, right out of the container) be brought to her with a spoon upon her arrival in the dining hall, because we knew that she would eat it. Although this plan of action was promised to our family, and the one "test" with me there worked fine, subsequent visits to the dining room confirmed that no yogurt was brought to her and that she was eating little to none of the regular food. I never was able to discover what the problem was—if there never had been a notation made to serve my mother the yogurt, or if the ever changing staff didn't know where to look for specific instructions, or if the staff simply didn't care enough to follow the instructions. I came to the conclusion that the nursing home food director and the nursing home administrator were not interested in complying with a care plan that required a specific action for a resident, no matter how ill the resident or how easy the request was to fulfill.

Nursing homes are often quite dry environments, especially in the winter when the air is naturally dry. I had asked the staff on a number of occasions to make sure that a glass of water be left on the table near my mother's reading chair, but I could not seem to get anyone's attention to remedy this situation. A few months later, the state sent a team of people to evaluate this nursing home, and they cited the nursing home for repeatedly ignoring the regulation that requires offering a beverage and snack to residents during the evening; they reported that they had not observed staff offering beverages to residents in the evening on any of the evenings that they were there.

Pool Staff and Other Staffing Problems

Many nursing homes avoid the high cost of full-time employees by hiring per diem (day at a time) or agency (also known as "pool") staff, particularly for evening, overnight, and weekend shifts. This constantly changing workforce cannot possibly get to know the residents enough to find out their preferences, nor do they necessarily take the time to read and follow existing care plans that could help them to do so.

The standard terminology used in nursing homes concerning resident care lays bare the impersonal nature of the care that is given: "Who is doing Mary Smith tonight?" you will hear one certified nursing assistant (CNA) ask another CNA. "I don't know, but I'm not doing her" will be a common response. "Doing (someone)" is language that is unacceptable to me. It indicates a very mechanical way of providing care. It also indicates that each staff member has a set list of residents that she will assist. This is very problematic, because if a resident is begging for help, she must wait until the staff member who is assigned to her is ready and willing to help.

On one occasion, a pool staff member came to help my mother get ready for bed. She came out of the bathroom with my mother wearing a flimsy hospital gown that was tied in the back, and then cranked up the head of her bed to about a 45 degree level. I asked her why she had done either of those things, since my mother had her own nightgowns and always slept on her side on a flat bed. She said "I always do this for everybody." I asked if she knew my mother's name or if she had read her care plan, and she said, "No, I don't have time to read care plans."

On other occasions, I found that pool staff had mistaken my mother for another resident with the same first name and were following the wrong care plan without realizing that they were doing so. Not even a simple quality control step of asking the resident "Are you Mrs. So and So?" was being followed. The lack of consistency in my mother's and other residents' care, and outright errors, were obvious to me and to a few other grown children who came in the evening to care for their parents.

We reported some errors, and long response times, to the nursing home administrator. When the situation failed to improve, I began to log my own notes concerning staffing levels each night, to see if there was a correlation between errors or long response times and staffing levels. My efforts to collect staffing data and correlate it with errors were completely blocked when the head nursing supervisor made a decision to post only aggregate staffing for the entire facility, not by floor, as had been done in the past. This direct attempt to stop my analysis based on data made me realize that the nursing home administration did not want to know if staffing levels were related to the frequency of mistakes. It was then that I began to realize that the only supervisor of quality control for my mother's care on the evening shift would be me.

Questionable Safety of Patients

When my family looked into the idea of placing my mother in a residential facility, one appealing aspect of the marketing materials was that the facility would offer a higher degree of safety than we could offer at home, especially since our mother had already taken one fall. The materials mentioned that residents' doors were left open at night so that safety checks could be done every fifteen minutes. The fear of liability lawsuits, particularly for falls, is the driving force behind most policies and procedures in nursing homes. This fear causes nursing homes to confine most residents to alarm-rigged wheelchairs except for a half-hour to hour of physical or occupational therapy a day. This restriction of movement is deemed to be necessary in order to achieve a high level of safety.

The restriction of an alarmed tether or pressure pad alarm in place is supposed to make it impossible for the resident to stand, let alone walk, without someone knowing that they are in danger. However, on many occasions when I visited my mother in the evening, alarm bells were going off and residents who were "fall risks" were staggering in their rooms or even down the hallway, without any staff in the vicinity to hear the alarm bell or see the danger to the resident. Since most residents of nursing homes (even non-dementia units) are too mentally and physically impaired to call for help if a loud alarm bell has been activated, and most nursing homes are inadequately staffed in the evening, even the residents supposedly being watched to prevent falls are vulnerable to life-threatening spills.

Over the course of a year, I observed many incidents where alarm bells would sound and stay ringing for ten or more minutes. I would have to leave my own mother to go searching the halls to try to find a staff person, since no staff were within eyesight or earshot. When I reported such concerns to the administration, I was told that the nursing home was within legal requirements for staffing, and nothing more could be done.

It finally came to pass that my mother left her alarmed bed and fell on the linoleum floor during a winter night. The nursing home could give us no information about how long she had been lying on the cold floor before someone finally found her. This also laid bare the marketing claim that residents are checked every fifteen minutes throughout the day and night.

On other separate occasions, I saw additional failures of safety protocols: I found my mother's heart pill in her bed (although it was recorded as having been administered by a nurse); a foil packet of A & D ointment on the floor next to her bed, where she (or I) could have slipped on it; a chemical-soaked cleaning rag in her bed, right next to her bed pillow; and large, razor-sharp shards of a broken mug in her nightstand table. Since only some of the pieces of the mug were there, someone on the staff must have known that a mug had broken, yet they had either failed to look for the other pieces, or even worse, had intentionally placed them there. It was a miracle that I did not cut my hand or wrist when I opened her nightstand table drawer to find a pen in her darkened room. These errors took place in a nursing home that prided itself as being one of the best in the United States, and which charged $8,000 a month for individual care. I came to realize, over the course of her year and a half in the nursing home, that the promise of safety was greatly exaggerated.

I look back on a very different scenario that happened with a neighbor of mine, one that points to a very different trajectory for living out one's life. A woman on my street had only one daughter, who married a man living abroad and raised her family there. After her husband died, this elderly woman made up her mind that she wanted to stay in her home, knowing full well that some day she would die, and probably die alone. She had daily contact with her neighbor across the street, a woman who knew her wishes about staying at home. This neighbor expected that some day she would not see the shades pulled up in the windows of the house across the street. That is exactly what happened, and that day she found her neighbor dead in her home at the age of 94. Until that day, she lived her life as she wished to live it, with joy and a great deal of independence, along with some respectful help from caring neighbors and friends.

Infection Control

The other factor that is certainly not mentioned to prospective visitors is a lack of infection control. It is not surprising, when considering that most nursing home residents have some degree of dementia, that most residents cannot remember to cover their mouths or noses when coughing or sneezing. What is surprising is that no protocols were in place to keep residents with coughs or colds segregated from healthy residents until they were not infectious. This means that upper respiratory illnesses passed through the nursing home population several times a year.

It is also not surprising that demented residents who self-toilet are probably not adequately washing their hands after using the toilet. *In the upscale nursing home in which my mother lived, there was no protocol or procedure about having residents wash their hands (or use an antibacterial hand spray) before entering the dining room and picking up and eating their food. Consequently, a gastrointestinal virus swept through the nursing home several times each year, causing severe diarrhea and immense suffering among the residents. The nursing home administration took a "there's nothing that we can do about it" stance to these infection control issues.*

If you think that I am being too harsh in my evaluation of this nursing home (one that claims to have one of the highest ratings in the U.S.), I should tell you that the state evaluation team found numerous deficits in its evaluation of the nursing home while my mother was there, including some of the issues that I had reported. Yet, even after the state cited the nursing home, the staff continued to verbalize a defiant attitude of denial, with one staff member saying, "If we had gotten the same team that we had the last year, we would have gotten a perfect score."

Loss of Physical Strength

As I have previously mentioned, the overriding concern of nursing home administrators is avoidance of liability lawsuits. Once a resident has a fall, they are deemed a "fall risk" and then are tethered to a wheelchair or chair, rather than being allowed to move about on their own accord. This is the "point of no return" for many elderly residents, for once their ability to walk is severely restricted throughout the day except for a brief period of physical and/or occupational therapy (usually only provided for 30-60 minutes, once or twice a day, five or six days a week), or a brief walk to the dining room and back, the resident begins to lose muscle mass and tone. This increases the risk of losing one's sense of balance as well as losing core body strength and overall coordination.

In addition, once the resident is confined to a wheelchair, they will usually require the help of one or two staff to bring them to the toilet and back. Given the understaffing in most nursing facilities and the long response times for toileting residents, it is only a matter of time before wheelchair-bound residents are put into the adult equivalent of diapers (Depends or other brands) to "prevent accidents."

Women who are diapered are especially prone to frequent urinary tract infections due to the transmission of fecal bacteria to the urinary tract, even when proper urinary/genital and anal care is meticulously done. *I found that many of the staff in the nursing home performed only cursory perineal care with my mother. When I inquired about the protocol for such care, and observed such care being done with my mother, I observed that the protocol being followed was such that it could easily transmit fecal matter to the urinary area. It was not a surprise, therefore, that my mother and other residents experienced debilitating episodes of urinary tract infections.*

It is important to note that elderly persons may not feel a burning sensation upon urinating that is a classic symptom in younger people with urinary tract infections. More often, lethargy and/or withdrawal and disinterest in eating are the presenting symptoms, not pain or burning. *There were several times when I was the one to bring these symptoms to the attention of the staff. If I had not been there to see them, no one would have noticed marked changes in her personality or eating habits.*

Increase in Psychological Problems

Psychological changes related to the restriction of movement in the elderly include loss of self-esteem, frustration, and anger. It erodes a person's dignity to have to beg to be taken to the bathroom and then wait a long time to be helped, or be lied to about how long it will take before help arrives. When a person who has always been able to use the toilet by themselves has to urinate in a diaper due to not being able to wait until help arrives, frustration, anger, disappointment and low self-esteem can all occur. The cumulative result of negative interactions with staff about toileting issues and other issues of control (such as not being able to go to bed at the desired time) often leads to "acting out" behavior. Unfortunately, many nursing homes and dementia care units do not address the underlying staffing shortages but instead medicate residents with psychotropic medications.

It is no wonder that the average life expectancy of people admitted to nursing facilities is two years. Infections, loss of mobility and health, and psychological problems are an endemic part of nursing home settings. Families beware—nursing home facilities are not designed or operated in a way to promote the health and wellness of residents. They are struggling institutions that are designed to limit legal liability and reduce overhead costs.

"Do unto others as you would have them do unto you," is the highest principle a family member can follow in thinking about whether nursing home care or home care would be in the dying person's best interest. Imagine yourself in a diaper in a wheel chair, having to wait for someone to take you to use a toilet, and ask yourself if that is what you wish for in your final months and days. If not, do you want to subject someone you love to those conditions?

If a Nursing Home is the Only or the Best Choice

I believe that at home or in-hospice care generally offers a higher quality of life for a dying person, and they should be the options of choice, if finances and family support are adequate. If your loved one chooses to live in a nursing home, or you make that decision for him, there are several ways in which you can ensure that your loved one will have the highest quality of life possible under those circumstances.

The most important thing that you and other family members can do is to visit as often as you possibly can, preferably daily. The personal contact that you have with your loved one will be the most meaningful minutes (or hours) of her day. For this reason, I encourage you to talk with your family members about which person is going to make the commitment to visit most frequently, and choose a nursing home that is most convenient for that person. It will make a world of difference to your loved one if you, or another "primary caregiver," will come by once a day, or even more often, rather than having days, weeks, or months go by without your loved one actually being with a close relative or friend.

How close should the nursing home be from the primary caregiver? That is something that you must decide based on your schedule and your willingness and ability to travel.

For me, I wanted my mother to be in a nursing home located very close to my workplace so that I could easily go to see her before or after work each day and I would have only a 20-25 minute drive each way to see her on the weekend. If the nursing home had not been near my work, and the drive each way had been longer, it would have been much more stressful for me to be there for her on a daily basis.

There is a feeling of abandonment that sets in for an elder when he is moved into an institutional setting, and this feeling deepens if he is only visited around the major holidays, when the parties are thrown for residents' families. Frequent visits by you and other family members will remind your father that he is deeply loved, even if he cannot be living in his home or in yours.

I can still remember the expressions on the faces of residents whose families did not come often, when they saw me come to visit my mother each day. They appreciated me coming and often said hello to me, yet underneath their desire to connect with me was also a sadness at the reality of their own lives, of weeks and months going by without face to face contact with children and grandchildren who lived far away, or—even harder to understand—those living close by but simply too busy to make the time to come.

If your loved one has any dementia, you have probably noticed the loss of their short term memory, of not being able to remember things from moment to moment or asking the same question over and over. One of the most difficult consequences of the brain-changing diseases of dementia and Alzheimer's disease is that when short term memory fades, the capacity to form new friendships is taken away. The formation of friendships depends upon one's ability to store and remember someone's name, physical characteristics, stories, interests, likes and dislikes, and other information that is essentially a "memory file" for the friend. If someone can no longer remember these things about the people around them, then they might as well be living in the middle of Grand Central Station, for they experience only a swirl of activity by the strangers around them.

Even though my mother was cogent enough to do her crossword puzzles and speak to me about our shared past experiences, she had lost her short term memory. She would glance over at her roommate on the other side of the room, put up her hand on the side toward her roommate, and then point at her palm and whisper, "Who is that?" I would whisper to her, "That is Jill, Mom. She's your roommate." "Oh," she would say, and she would nod her head up and down. This was a regular conversation that we had, even after my mother had shared her nursing home room with Jill for a full year. It became evident to me that my mother was not capable of forming any relationships with caregivers, since she could not retain any information about even the woman with whom she shared a room after a year of living with her.

As the months went on, my mother's short term memory could no longer even register when I or my family members had visited. Once, I saw a close relative walk out of my mother's room. When I went in to see her, I mentioned seeing him, and she said, "I haven't seen him in a very long time." However, even though I am certain that she could not remember when I had just visited with her, either, my mother was always very grateful when I was with her and that is all that mattered to me, for I knew that in those moments of connection, my mother felt loved.

Quality at the End of Life Depends on Time Spent with Your Loved One

This is the most important concept that I can share with you: quality of life at the end of life is all about family members (however you define them) spending time with your loved one. Only you who know and love him will remember the stories and memories that are still inside his mind, and you can relive those memories and stories with him. These story telling sessions make meaning for an elderly person when their present reality has no meaning because they have no remembrance of history or connection to the people around them.

Even competent, caring service by the best of trained staff cannot compensate for the lack of personal contact with close relatives or friends. While phone calls and letters are certainly better than having no contact, hearing one's young granddaughter on the phone will never replace getting a hug around the neck from her, or having her come to sit in grandpa's lap and show him her new picture book. Likewise, a grown daughter's gesture of stroking her mother's hand or running her fingers through her mother's hair is priceless to the elderly or dying person.

Form Relationships with Nursing Home Staff

Visiting often and at different times of day is important for another reason, too, so that you get to know the people who work on each shift and you become knowledgeable about the services that the facility provides. I encourage you to take the time to introduce yourself to the certified nursing assistants (CNAs) and the registered nurses and licensed practical nurses (RNs and PNs) on at least the day and evening shifts. It is helpful to bring a small notebook with you for recording their names, so that you can remember them when you see them next.

Establishing a friendly relationship with the CNAs and nurses will be very beneficial in several ways: First, if they realize that you are an advocate who is dedicated to ensuring the quality of care for your loved one, they will be likely to really notice what is going on for your loved one and talk with you first- hand about changes in his condition when you visit. Second, by getting to know the CNAs, and appreciating the work that they do, you will help to lift the morale of these lowly paid, overworked and underappreciated helpers.

It is a sad fact that our society pays workers very poorly who work with the most vulnerable populations among us—young children and the very elderly. These are the two groups who are literally without voices, who are either too young to formulate the ideas to express themselves or too infirm, physically and mentally, to be able to speak about their needs and advocate for themselves. Taking the time to compliment someone for their energy, enthusiasm, helpfulness or dedication to their work will lift their spirits and give them a sense that they are valued.

I also encourage you to be as helpful as you are able to be, by visiting with other residents, responding to your loved one's requests for assistance, and being willing to lend a helping hand with your loved one's care when a staff member calls in sick at the last minute. The staff grew to respect me, as I respected them, when they saw that I was not above doing the "hands on" work of personal care with my mother. Sometimes, having to care for one fewer resident, on a short staffed busy evening, made all of the difference to the CNA, as well as ensuring that my mother would be cleaned up and in bed by 9:30 pm.

Form a Self-Help Support Network of Family Caregivers

Be sure to introduce yourself to family caregivers whom you see taking care of their relatives. If you share your name and telephone number or email address with the families of other persons in the same nursing home, you will be able to form a network of support among family members who are caregivers. By doing so, you will likely discover that you are all experiencing similar problems. There is strength in numbers, and while your attempts to address problems may not always be met with an attitude of helpfulness or with actual success on the part of the nursing home administrator, if you approach the administration as a group of concerned families, your reports of problems will probably be given greater credence.

Change Comes, Though Slowly

Even though many of our reports of problems were not addressed as we had hoped, we did manage to make some progress in having the nursing home make changes, both major and minor. One of our support group's requests, that a television be placed in the lounge area on the nursing home wing so that residents wouldn't just be sitting in their wheelchairs in a silent lounge area for hours at a time, waiting to be put to bed in the evening, was roundly rejected by the nursing home social worker, who commented that if we wanted a television we should go out and buy one ourselves. However, a few months later, a large screen television was installed in that lounge.

Another one of our concerns was that it was often impossible for us to locate a CNA during the evening shift if our family member, or another resident, needed help. It became obvious to us that even the CNAs could not find out where the other CNAs were at any given time, because they were usually behind closed bathroom doors helping residents and because there was no intercom or pager system to send messages to staff or between staff. This concern, relayed several times to the nursing home administrator, was dismissed with statements about the fact that the nursing home was meeting or exceeding the state mandated staffing requirements. However, by the time that my mother left that facility, the nursing home was in the process of testing a pager system that would allow CNAs and nurses to communicate with each other.

Change in any institution is slow and difficult, and nursing homes are no exception. I have come to believe, however, that nursing homes need the advocacy of family groups to encourage them to change for the better, and when encouragement isn't enough, family groups should insist that they make improvements, for the safety and wellbeing of all residents.

One of my relatives was reluctant to bring up safety issues if they didn't directly relate to my mother. I pointed out that if Mrs. Doe is staggering down the hall, with her alarm bell going off but no one around to hear it or respond, it could be my mother staggering down the hall in the weeks or months to follow.

It is truly the case that it takes a village to care for an elder, and having a cooperative group of caregivers who keep an eye out for each others' loved ones and advocate for the wellbeing of all residents is both a necessary safety net and a needed source of support for family caregivers.

CHAPTER NINE

FINANCIAL CONSIDERATIONS

- Costs of At Home Care
- Costs of Assisted Living Care
- Costs of Nursing Home Care
- Costs of Hospice Care
- Planning Ahead for Medicare and Medicaid
- Long Term Care Insurance – Pros and Cons

Making the decision about whether to die at home, to move in with a relative or friend, or to move to a nursing facility or live-in hospice is a decision that is complicated for many reasons, including financial reasons.

The most major factor in the overall cost of personal care is the amount of nursing care (registered nurse or practical nurse), certified nursing assistant care, or family/friend (volunteer) caregiving that is needed and is available. Other factors include whether the person has dementia or mental illness (and what type and to what degree), whether the person's medical condition requires specialized equipment, and whether the person's weight or medical condition requires two caregivers at once to turn the person in their bed, or to feed, bathe, assist with toileting activities, or administer treatments to them.

Costs of At Home Care

The cost of at home care can range significantly, depending on the level of care needed and whether the person needs part-time or full-time care. In addition, the cost per hour of skilled certified nursing assistant care, licensed practical nursing care, or registered nursing care, varies considerably from region to region, or even within a region. This is why it is important to interview a number of providers, to find out what services are offered at what cost per hour, and the minimum number of hours of care that can be scheduled at a time.

Costs of Assisted Living Care

The cost per month of assisted living can range from $1,500 to $4,500 or more per month. In addition, many assisted facilities also require the payment of an upfront sum that can be thousands, to tens of thousands, of dollars. The monthly cost of assisted living care is not Medicare reimbursable.

In some facilities, part or all of the upfront payment is refundable on a prorated, declining balance basis, should the resident not remain in the assisted living unit for the minimum period of time specified in the refund clause of the contract. It is very important to read all of the fine print in such contracts!

If the assisted living resident's health status changes for the worse and the person is required to move to a skilled nursing facility, unless the person has met the Medicare qualifications of having a three day hospitalization, the family may need to pay the monthly rate for the skilled nursing facility (see the costs of nursing home care below).

Costs of Nursing Home Care

The cost of living in a private nursing home can range from $5,000 to $15,000 or more per month, depending on the type of facility, the services it offers, the number of residents per room, and where the facility is located. It is important to note that some nursing homes are "private pay" only. Even with nursing homes that accept Medicare, the cost of nursing home care is covered by Medicare only if certain criteria are met and for a limited time period.

Costs of Hospice Care

Generally, hospice care is covered by Medicare and private insurance. However, the types of services and quantity of care provided by hospices in different states varies enormously. To find out what local hospice organizations provide under Medicare or your private insurance, contact the local hospices in your area directly or call your insurance provider.

One of the hopeful signs that I see on the horizon is that legislation is being considered and voted on in several states to shift more funding to at home hospice care, which would increase the options for more families to keep their loved ones at home in the final chapters of their lives.

Planning Ahead for Medicare and Medicaid

If you think that your loved one will eventually need to live in a nursing home, you will want to learn as much as possible about Medicare and Medicaid regulations. The first step is to go to www.medicare.gov or to call the toll free number listed on page 163 under "Medicare" to learn about these governmental programs.

I also suggest that you consider consulting with a lawyer who is skilled in Medicare and Medicaid laws, in order to receive specific advice concerning your family's financial assets and estate plans. Many people do not realize how difficult it is to qualify for governmentally-subsidized nursing home care, and they also are not aware of the many regulations concerning what assets can be kept and which must be spent down before Medicaid eligibility begins. It is better to become aware of the regulations regarding these programs now, rather than wait and be told that you are ineligible in the midst of a health crisis.

Long Term Care Insurance—Pros and Cons

The long term care insurance industry is a relatively young industry, and it remains to be seen whether the products being marketed now will live up to their promises in decades to come. If you do decide to investigate long term care policies, please do not act impulsively to purchase a product after your first conversation with a convincing sales person. The purchase of long term care insurance is a major investment of your resources, and you will want to be sure that you have purchased a plan that will meet your needs without bankrupting you in the process. Take the time to meet with representatives from several companies; compare the benefits and costs of different plans; and investigate, through research, the ratings of the companies offering the plans.

Those who favor long term care insurance, including many state governments, feel that Medicare and Medicaid will be unlikely to be able to fund eldercare in the coming decades and therefore private long term care insurance is an important part of the solution.

Those who are skeptical about long term care insurance point to the fact that longevity tables for the large baby boom generation are still hypothetical. While elderly persons who have paid long term care insurance premiums for decades are now able to draw full benefits from their policies, no one can determine if the accrued payments by the baby boom generation will be able to sustain the burgeoning numbers of persons who will be drawing on those benefits in decades to come.

If you do look into long term care insurance, consider whether the plan will be inflation protected, in other words, that its purchasing power today will maintain its current value two or three decades from now. Also look for flexibility in paying equal benefits for at home or nursing home care. Having a policy that will only partially cover at home care when you need it twenty years from now will not be sufficient unless you have significant financial resources to make up the difference in expenses.

CHAPTER TEN

SIX SURPRISES ABOUT
THE DYING PROCESS

- Dress Rehearsals for Dying (False Alarms)
- The Flickering of the Flame
- Animals Know Before We Do
- Communicating with the Beyond
- The Spiritual Aspect of Witnessing Someone Die
- Medical Surprises

Dying is not a predictable process, although certain illnesses have distinct phases of progression. If you wish to educate yourself about the medical aspects of the progression of a specific illness, I encourage you to read *How We Die* by Sherwin B. Nuland (see page 164) and to consult web sites listed for specific conditions, some of which are listed in the resource listings on pages 157–166.

Each of the persons I have helped in the final phases of their lives died in their own way and in their own time, just as each lived his or her life in a unique way. While acknowledging the uniqueness of the journey for each dying person, I will point out six surprising elements that I, or one of my friends, experienced as a loved one declined in health. These may or may not happen in your loved one's journey toward the end of this life, but you may find it helpful to be aware of the possibility of encountering them.

Dress Rehearsals for Dying (False Alarms)

In these situations, the person has had a dramatic turn for the worse in their medical status, bringing them to the brink of dying. Then, remarkably, they have bounced back and recovered enough to leave the crisis phase and reach a place of stability. I have found that these dress rehearsals have also happened with pets that I have had. These episodes can be alarming, but each instance has made me face my loved one's mortality in a direct way and has helped me to prepare for what was to come.

The Flickering of the Flame

The second surprising thing that I have noticed is that in two instances, my loved ones had what I refer to as the *flickering of the candle flame*, a period of increased vitality within a day or two of dying. This was most pronounced in the case of my father, who was struggling with the final stages of lung and heart disease. *The day before he died, I called a beloved cousin to say that if she wanted to see my father one more time, she should come the next day. To my great surprise, my father was energetic and animated on that day—telling stories, laughing and thoroughly enjoying her visit. I looked at him as they laughed and talked and thought, "Well, maybe he isn't dying after all!" By the next morning, the flame of life was barely there, and he breathed his last breath before noon.* In the process of researching this book, I have seen the phenomenon of increased vitality within a day or two of death mentioned on several hospice websites, so it is not unique to my loved ones' journeys.

Animals Know Before We Do

I had read years ago about a cat in a nursing home who had the uncanny ability to know when someone was going to die. In the article, the nurses said that they always knew when someone would die, because the cat would be drawn to that person and wouldn't leave their side until their death.

When my mother was transferred from the nursing unit to the dementia unit, I noticed that there were two gray cats on that unit, neither of which appeared to like spending time with people. They usually stayed by themselves or played in the halls late at night. I asked one of the nurses if the cats knew when people were going to die. She said, "Absolutely." About four months later, my mother's health declined rapidly, and we were called on a Monday morning to be told that her blood oxygen was in the high 70s, and she was unresponsive. When I entered her room, I saw the two cats sitting there, near her bed. This told me that her time was nearing. Even though some of the nurses said that they did not feel that she would die soon, I decided to stay with her for the next few days. During those two days, the two cats walked around her bed, kept jumping up on her bed, and came to sit in my lap (which they had never attempted to do before). They hardly left her room. My mother died at 4 am on that Wednesday morning, with me by her side. Within minutes of her death, both of the gray boy cats strolled out of the room, as if to state, "That job is done."

Communicating with the Beyond

Another surprise that I had was that two of my dying relatives seemed to have communication with deceased relatives in the months or days before they died.

Four months before my mother's death, while she was sitting in her chair doing crossword puzzles, she told my sister that my father (deceased for seven years) had just left her nursing home room and he was gone to play golf. When I saw her an hour or so later, she said the same thing to me. I asked if she knew with whom he was playing golf, she said he was with a man but she didn't know his name. She seemed very matter of fact about it, as if he had just walked out of the room, even though she consciously knew that he was deceased.

Seventeen years prior, when I was staying with my grandmother in her final week of life, I heard her talking in the middle of the night. I went into her room to see her sitting up (which she had not done in many days), looking up to the ceiling and holding up her hands, and speaking to her departed husband. She was excitedly speaking to him, and addressing him by name, although I could not make out the content of what she was saying. She seemed to be totally in an altered state and when I addressed her, she ignored me. After completing her conversation with my deceased grandfather, she lay back down and went immediately to sleep. When I questioned her about it the next morning, she had no recollection of having sat up in bed or having talked with my grandfather.

The Spiritual Aspect of Witnessing Someone Die

My fifth surprise is that I have felt a strong sense of a spiritual experience on two occasions being with dying people.

Right before my grandmother died, I sensed her energy withdrawing from her limbs and torso, into her forehead area. It was as if she were intensely thinking about something important. Then, at the moment of her death, I sensed (rather than saw) her spirit exit her body out of the top of her head, and then felt it hover near the ceiling of her room, above her head, as if her soul were looking down on her body and on a relative and me, saying "I can't believe I did it—I'm no longer in my body." My relative also sensed her spirit there above us, so we continued to talk to her spirit and tell her that, yes, she had left her body, but she could stay there as long as she needed to, before going on to the next journey. I continued to sit with her body and talk and sing to her spirit until, all of a sudden, her spirit was gone, as if rocket propelled, to somewhere far away.

My sibling and I had a different experience at the death of my father, but one that was equally powerful. My father had always said that he was a "devout atheist." However, at the moment of death, he had what I can only imagine was a spiritual experience. As he passed the threshold from life to death, a look of joy, awe, and amazement come over his face, as if he had just seen something very beautiful and awe-inspiring. This was quite startling to me, given his beliefs about simply returning "dust to dust."

Different religions have very different teachings concerning death and the afterlife. If your loved one has a particular religious viewpoint, consulting his or her clergyperson for information concerning this topic may be appropriate, or you may be interested in exploring book and web resources on near-death experiences in the resource chapter on page 164.

Medical Surprises

The last surprises are more of a medical nature. One happened not to me, but to a friend giving care to his father:

His elderly father had had a pacemaker inserted into his chest years before, to keep his heart beating regularly. Although he had questioned his father's cardiologist about what might happen at the time of death, given that he had a pacemaker, the cardiologist could not, or would not, give him any clear answers.

What my friend relayed to me, a few months after his father's death, was that the pacemaker caused a very traumatic situation for his father, his mother, and him. His father was at the point of death, and just as he had stopped breathing and they thought he had died, the pacemaker kicked back in and jolted him back to life, causing him to struggle and gasp for breath. After struggling several moments, he once again collapsed into what seemed like his final moment of life. Once again, the pacemaker kicked in, jolting him back to life and causing him to struggle for breath. This gruesome sequence happened three times before the pacemaker finally gave up, emitting a loud, solid tone, and then shut off.

What could have been a quiet, good death ended up being fraught with stress and anguish for all concerned, due to not having been properly informed about how the pacemaker would function as he died. If your loved one has a pacemaker, I recommend that you directly address this particular issue with the hospice team (as well as the doctor) to receive advice and counseling concerning what options you and your loved one have concerning his pacemaker's operation.

Note: It is very important to inform the funeral director if the dying person has a pacemaker and you wish to have their body cremated. The pacemaker must be removed before cremation or it can cause a dangerous explosion that could inflict damage or death on the cremation center staff.

The other medical surprise that I wish to mention, and which I observed, was having to contend with a state of "terminal agitation" in a loved one during her last day of life. Normally a quiet, very acquiescent person, she became extremely agitated to the point of being out of control. Although she had no strength and could no longer stand, she kept trying to crawl out of her bed, in a state of fear and delusion, although she didn't know where she wanted to go. She kept yelling, "Don't leave me" even though we were with her and we told her again and again that we would not leave her. She also became so hot that she could not stand having any clothes on, something that was the opposite from her normal desire to be wrapped in warm clothes and a sweater.

This is where the expertise and skill of the hospice staff is invaluable. We made a call to the hospice nurse, who knew exactly what this "terminal agitation" was, and within 20 minutes, the nurse was there to assess the situation, firsthand, and then to consult with the physician by phone so that he could adjust her medication. Thanks to their knowledge and skills, my wonderful relative was able to be calm and peaceful in the last day of her life, and she died with me by her side.

CHAPTER ELEVEN

THE FINAL DAYS, HOURS, AND MINUTES

- Telling Someone That They Are Dying, or Not?
- What Do Dying People Eat?
- Music and Dying
- Watchful Witnessing and Pain Management Decisions
- Physical Changes
- Saying What You Need to Say
- Being Present at the Moment of Death and Rituals to Consider
- If You Have to Wait for the Funeral Director to Arrive

Telling Someone That They Are Dying, or Not?

When I think about the final stages of dying, the phrase "this durable, fragile thing called life" keeps coming to me. This is because dying is not a strictly linear process, and it can have unexpected turns for the better or for the worse. I have been told by nurses and hospice nurses that they have seen some people die more quickly than they thought they would, and conversely, they have seen people hang on for months longer than they thought would be possible.

I do not advocate anyone telling someone that they have two months, four days, five hours and 47 minutes left to live, because that is not the kind of thing that anyone can predict with such accuracy. However, I personally believe that a person deserves to know if the end of his life is near. I have found that being truthful with someone at the end of his life can enable him to enter into a process of spiritual readiness, so that death can come peacefully. Unfortunately, some doctors and nurses are so afraid of losing a patient that they cannot bring themselves to face the reality of the condition of their patient, let alone discuss it with the patient.

Such was the case with one of my elderly friends. *I had gone to see her in the hospital, knowing that she had fallen in the nursing home and her vital signs were weak. I met her close friend and medical agent in the hall, who delivered the grim news that the scan had revealed a huge mass in her abdomen and internal bleeding, and there was nothing more to be done. She would die in a matter of hours or, at most, days. I asked if the doctor or anyone had talked with her about this. She said, "Yes, but he talked to her while she was sleeping." I asked if she wanted to be the one to deliver the news to our mutual friend, but she declined, saying that she was too overcome with emotion to do so.*

I realized that this task was up to me. I went to her bedside and sat with her until her eyes opened. Then, I stood very close to her face and greeted her and held her hand. I said, "I am very sorry, but I have some bad news to give you. The results of the scan came back and they show that you have a very large mass in your abdomen, and you are bleeding internally. There is nothing more that the doctors can do for you, and you will probably die in the next day or two. I will be here as much as I can, so if you want to die with me here with you, I will be honored to witness your passing. If you want to die alone, I will also give you time alone so that you can decide to die with your privacy, if that is what you wish."

This dear friend, who had not been able to speak for months, fixed her eyes on mine, and then, after a strong sigh, said "Oh well," with her characteristic resonant, deep voice. I put my check against hers, and told her how very much I cared for her and I thanked her for the conversations that we had shared, talking about current world situations over cups of tea. I sat with her late into the evening, and after she had been asleep for several hours, I went home to rest for a few hours. The next morning I received a call saying that she had died some time during the night. I felt a deep sense of peace at having allowed her to know that her time had come.

A friend of mine told me a wonderful story about helping to care for a male friend of hers. As he was getting very near the end of his life, she went to see him in the nursing home. Another friend was leaving his room just as she was coming in. He said to her, "You had better say something, he is really struggling and won't let go."

Knowing that her friend had spent a lot of his life working in the theater, she said to him in a celebratory tone of voice, "The performance is over, the house lights are coming up, and the audience is applauding. They loved it! You've taken your final bow. Now it is time to leave the stage." His eyelids flickered and he died about 45 minutes later.

Of course, the decision to talk about death is a very personal decision to be made by the dying persons' caregivers, in light of knowing the dying person and thinking about whether the person would want to know about their impending death, or not.

Another close friend of mine cared for her mother in her mother's home. My friend attempted to talk with her mother about her wishes for end of life care, but each time she did, her mother refused to discuss anything about death or dying. My friend referred to her mother as a "death denier." Her mother continued to deny that she was dying right through to the end, and refused to talk about planning for her funeral arrangements. My friend realized that this was what her mother wanted, and that she and her sister would have to make the decisions about end of life care and funeral arrangements on their own.

If your loved one does not wish to talk to you about the fact that she is dying, it is best to respect her wishes to not discuss these subjects. It is also a good idea not to discuss these topics in her presence, even if she appears to be sleeping or is in a coma. Medical research has documented many cases where people in comas have come back to consciousness and have reported their frustration and/or anger at having heard medical staff or family members saying things to which they would have objected if they had been able to respond at the time.

What Do Dying People Eat?

It is often the case that in the last weeks or days of life, the dying person's desire for food begins to wane and the person may eat or drink less, or may even stop eating and drinking altogether. On the other hand, the dying person may have a sudden resurgence of interest in food, or perhaps in specific foods.

When my grandmother was in her final week of life, and had not eaten for two days, she suddenly asked a relative, "What do dying people eat?" The relative replied, "Anything they want to eat,

Gramma." She then said she would like a large bowl of soft serve va-
nilla ice cream, which my relative went out and bought for her, and
which she consumed with gusto. It was the last true meal that she en-
joyed, and she really did enjoy it.

I have another set of friends whose mother had been refusing to eat
the food at the nursing home, believing that it was causing her gas-
trointestinal problems. She was having more and more conflicts with
the staff, who kept putting spoonfuls of food into her mouth, even
when she would say "No!" Shortly thereafter, they moved her from the
nursing home to a live-in hospice, a wonderful place that allowed resi-
dents to eat anything that they wanted to eat, whenever they wanted
to eat it. In this more respectful environment, their mother began eat-
ing heartily again, consuming large bowls of beef stew and other
made-to-order foods that she enjoyed. Her last months were happy
ones because she had the control over what she ate, and when and
where she ate it, and she was able to enjoy her peaceful, private room
in a very quiet setting.

Music and Dying

Music has a powerful capacity to evoke memories of the past. If
your dying parent, spouse, partner or friend liked to listen to particular types of music or to particular performers, then I encourage
you to think about playing the music that she loved, even if it is not
music to which you would choose to listen.

If you are using the services of a hospice or a cancer support organization, you might ask the staff if they know of any live performers who are willing to come to play at the homes of dying persons on
a pro bono (voluntary) or fee-based basis. There are certain musi-
cians who dedicate part or all of their performing hours to easing
the way of persons who are dying by playing soothing music and/or
music of particular religious traditions. (See Music Thanatology
page 163 and www.caringfordyinglovedones.com.)

In the case of my father, we knew that he loved hearing people sing-
ing in harmony, such as barbershop music, The Mills Brothers, Nat
King Cole, and certain gospel groups (even though he was an atheist!).
We played such music for him in his bedroom, knowing that on an in-
ner level he was singing along, since he knew all of the words by heart.

My friend's mother loved Cole Porter. Even at the end when she couldn't recognize her son or daughter because of her advanced Alzheimers disease, she would perk up upon hearing the CD, and even say some of the words. As my friend said, "The mind has the capacity to relate to music on a very deep level."

Watchful Witnessing and Pain Management Decisions

Once your loved one has entered an interior state of not being fully awake, or being partially awake but not being able to speak, you will need to read the clues as to whether he or she is in pain. Knowing her normal facial expressions, bodily postures, and vocal habits will be of great help to you. For example, if she never furrowed her brow, or ground her teeth, clenched her fists, or groaned, these could be signs of internal discomfort and pain that should be brought to the attention of the nurse or doctor.

Even if your loved one can talk to you, he might not admit being "in pain" even though he is experiencing pain. Pain is a word with which some people don't identify, or perhaps, he might see admission of pain as a sign of weakness. An example of this might be helpful.

The nurses on the unit in the nursing home where my mother lived for the last 4 months of her life insisted that my mother's groans were simply repetitive verbalizations due to her advancing dementia, because when they asked her if she was in pain, she would say, "No."

I tried my own experiment. When I asked her if she was in pain, she said, "No." Then I asked her if she was uncomfortable, and she said, "Yes, uncomfortable." When I then asked where she was uncomfortable, she would stroke and hold her distended belly.

You, as a person who knows the dying person, will have a better idea of how to talk to the person who is ill, in order to find out if pain might be part of his experience. When the dying person can no longer speak, all that you will have to go by is your experience of the person before and during her illness, as this next anecdote shows:

When my high school classmates all banded together to care for our 54 year old friend who was dying of pancreatic cancer, we used facial cues (furrowed brow and grimaces) to inform the hospice nurse when we felt that she was suffering and needed increased medication. In this way, we were able to alleviate her pain and enable her to die peacefully.

Physical Changes

As your loved one progresses toward death, you may begin to notice changes that can be mental, physical, or emotional in nature. These might include the tendency to withdraw from contact with you or with the outside world, changes in sleeping habits, weakening or loss of appetite, a rattling sound while breathing (or times when breathing ceases and then begins again), changes in the color of the feet or hands or other areas of the body, or a sense of your loved one being very cold or very hot.

Each person's dying process is very unique, so it is not possible to provide a map to follow in predicting what will happen, even within the course of a specific illness. If you wish to learn more about the physiological changes that take place during the final stages of illnesses such as cancer, stroke, heart disease, and AIDS, I recommend that you read *How We Die* by Sherwin D. Nuland. (See page 164.)

Saying What You Need to Say

Only you know what it is that you need to say to someone before they die. Perhaps you already know those words, or perhaps they will come to you as you sit with the dying person. I encourage you to trust your inner sense of what it is that you need to say to your dying loved one and express those sentiments before you cannot do so. I have had two experiences that have been profound in this regard:

In the case of caring for my father, my life partner and I cared for him in his home. Toward the very end of his life, I sensed that he was holding on because of a fear of not knowing if my mother would be taken care of. My partner and I sat by his bedside and I said, "Dad, it's OK for you to go. Jo and I will take care of Mom. We will do our very best to make sure that she has everything she needs. You have been a wonderful caregiver to her for 64 years, and now it is time to hand that over to us. You don't need to worry. We will take care of her from now on." He seemed to relax at that point, even though he couldn't speak, and he died the next morning.

In the case of caring for my mother, I was sitting with her in the depth of night, not knowing if she would die on my watch, or if she would live another day or two, or three. Sometime in that darkness, I felt the desire to tell her every memory that I could bring to mind about her caring for me, from my earliest recollections to the present time. I told her story after story, sometimes laughing and sometimes with tears streaming down my face, while she lay unconscious in the bed. I talked to her for hours, and then my life story with her was complete. Very shortly after I finished my last story, the CNAs came in to change her undergarments. I was looking closely at her, full of love for her and watching her breath go in and out, when her breathing simply stopped. There was no sound and no movement, only a look of profound peace that came over her face. It was a gentle passing from this life to the next, so gentle that I had to tell the CNAs to stop, that I believed she had just died.

I had no thought at the time that recounting my life with her would enable her to feel the completeness of her life story and move on to the great mystery of the afterlife, but that is what seemed to have happened that night.

I hope that you will trust yourself to say what you feel called to say to your loved one in her final hours. By doing so, you may assist her in making her transition.

Being Present at the Moment of Death and Rituals to Consider

No matter how much you expect your loved one to die, no matter how old he is or how much she has suffered, the moment of death ushers in a profound sense of loss for many people. It is up to you to determine what you need in order to honor your loved one and honor your own sense of grieving. Do not feel pressured by medical or nursing home staff to immediately vacate the room or have the deceased person's body removed from the room.

My own sense of what I wanted to do at and after the moment of death has changed during the past two decades. *In 1991, when I was with my grandmother at the time of her death, I knew that I wanted to sit with her body until her spirit had departed, but I had no concept of what should happen next, other than calling the funeral director. At the point that we felt her spirit had departed, we called the funeral di-*

rector, who came to put my grandmother's body on a gurney and take it to the funeral home.

Several years after my grandmother's death, a dear friend told me the story of how she went back to her native country of Lithuania in time to be present for her mother's death. She was kind enough to share the details with me of how she lovingly bathed her mother's body and clothed her in her chosen apparel, rather than allowing an undertaker to do this most intimate work. I shared this story with my sibling and we agreed that we would want to do this for each of our parents, if possible. In 2001, after our father died in his home in his bed, we played music and sang as we washed our father's body, shampooed his hair, and then put him into his favorite flannel pajamas, according to his wishes. This ritual bath was a powerful way for us to show our love and respect to him. In 2008, we did the same thing for our mother after she died, bathing her body in her nursing home room, and clothing her in her favorite blue silk dress, according to her wishes.

Prior to caring for each of my parents' bodies after they died, I had mistakenly thought that rigor mortis would immediately set in upon death and the body would become cold and inflexible. I was surprised to realize, when bathing my father's body, that his body stayed warm and flexible for quite a long time after his death, so it was not a difficult procedure to bathe him or put on his pajamas. There was a wonderful sense of us giving each of our parents a final gift by so carefully washing their skin and anointing it with fragrant lotion before clothing each of them for the last time.

I have experienced the time immediately after the death to be a profound time to be with the person who has died. The important thing is to trust yourself to feel whatever you are feeling, and to take the time that you need with your loved one before the funeral director moves their body. I have learned from a compassionate funeral director that it is also possible for family members to participate in other after-death rituals such as helping to lift the loved one's body from the bed onto the stretcher, or walking alongside the body as it is brought to the hearse. Not all families will want to share in such intimate tasks or intimate moments, but it is freeing to know that you can do so, if you wish.

If You Have to Wait for the Funeral Director to Arrive

It is important to realize that the funeral home director will not always be able to respond immediately to your call to come to get the body of your deceased loved one. *A funeral home director told me of one instance where he received a call from a family whose loved one had just died. At the moment of that call, he was attending a burial service and was about to assist at a different memorial service immediately following the burial, and his other staff members were driving to a location at some distance to receive a body. Therefore, he told them that he would not be able to come to pick up the body for several hours.*

Unfortunately, the nursing home administrator told the family that they could not legally leave the room with the body until the funeral home director came for the body. Without knowing their rights in a situation such as this (there is no law stating that you must stay in the room with the body of a deceased person until the funeral home director arrives) the family took the administrator's word as "the law," and several family members became emotionally distressed by not being able to leave the room for several hours.

If this situation should ever occur to you in a nursing home setting, it is important to know that you are not obligated to stay with the body of your loved one until the funeral director arrives. If you choose to stay, that is fine, but if you choose to leave, that is fine, too.

Note: it is important that the nurse in a hospital or nursing home fill out the "nurse pronouncement form" correctly, and with a black pen, following the death, to ensure that there will not be delays in securing certificates of death. You can ask to see that form, to make sure that the deceased person's name and other information is correct and that the form has been filled out with a black pen.

CHAPTER TWELVE

RIDING THE ROLLER COASTER OF GRIEF

- Beginning to Grieve Your Loved Ones
  Before They Are Gone
- Coping in the Days Following the Death
- Exhaustion, Disorientation, or Numbness
- Sadness, Anger, Aloneness, and Other
  Strong Emotions
- Feeling the Presence of Your Departed Loved One
- Honoring your Grieving Process

Beginning to Grieve Your Loved Ones Before They Are Gone

The grieving process can begin when your loved one dies, or it may begin much earlier. You may begin to grieve the loss of your loved one during the long, slow course of his illness, as every aspect of your relationship with him changes. If your loved one has dementia, you may feel an emotional impact not only due to his memory loss but also the personality changes that can attend dementia. These personality changes can result in complete role reversals: where you had formerly been a daughter, you become the parent. Or, if your spouse suffers from dementia, you may have to take on the roles that he had always held.

It is important for you to validate that you are experiencing grief at the loss of your loved one, even though they are still living. Persons who have never lost a loved one can be perplexed or even unsympathetic in response to sadness and grief expressed while your loved one is still alive. If you cannot find support among your friends or relatives, you will be able to do so by contacting organizations that are designed to support people in caring for dying persons. Your local hospice, as well as the American Cancer Society, the Alzheimer's Association, and other service organizations can provide volunteer and professional help to guide you through your grieving, whenever it occurs. (Please see pages 158 and 161.)

With internet websites being added by the thousands each day, searching on the word "grief" or "grieving" or "grief support groups" will yield many references for information or services related to grieving.

The process of grieving is as individual as the process of dying. The descriptions of phases of grieving listed below are meant to be helpful as you experience your own, very personal relationship to grieving, but you should not feel constrained by them. Whatever way you grieve is YOUR way and should be honored by you and the people who love you, unless you find that you are stuck somewhere along your path for an extended period of time in a way that feels unhealthy to you. In that case, reach out for professional assistance, for you might be suffering from clinical depression or another condition that can be eased by psychotherapy, group support, holistic therapies, or medication.

Coping in the Days Following the Death

If you have not done any preparation for funeral services, then the days following a death will be especially demanding, as you visit the funeral home, write an obituary, meet with a clergyperson, and make arrangements for a reception following the funeral.

You should not feel as if you have to hold the funeral on the day after your loved one dies unless your religious custom dictates a burial within a certain period of time. A funeral director told me that with modern facilities a body can be kept for up to 72 hours, even without embalming. Allowing yourself a slightly longer time frame to finalize your plans will allow family members from far away the time to travel to the services and it will also allow you some time for rest. This is important because the 24 hours during which the memorial service, funeral, and burial take place may be an intensely stressful time for you.

As you communicate with family members and friends, you will probably see that people deal with intense stress and grief in different ways. One member of the family might go into complete seclusion, overcome with emotion. Yet another might bury herself in work, as if nothing has happened. Another may drown his sorrow with alcohol or drugs.

You may be fortunate and have excellent cooperation between family members, or you may feel that your family is more dysfunctional than ever in this period of time. As with the caregiving phase, many of the duties of planning a funeral and memorial may fall to one person to fulfill, and that person may end up being you. If cooperation is not to be had within the family, be sure to enlist the support of close friends or a professional counselor or clergyperson to assist you in coping with the duties before you.

Note: Some people find it impossible to cry, although they are grieving. This may be deeply disturbing to them, as well as to family members who regard them as cold or heartless. If you cannot cry, talk to your loved ones about it so that they know that you are grieving, even if you cannot express it in the way that they do. If you feel that your emotions are all bottled up inside of you and you cannot gain access to them, consider talking to a counselor about ways to get in touch with your feelings.

Exhaustion, Disorientation, or Numbness

Especially if you have been the primary caregiver, you may find that following the wake, funeral or memorial service, you may feel exhausted, numb, or even disoriented. You have been in overdrive during the last final months or weeks of your loved one's illness, and you probably have deprived yourself of sleep in order to be at your loved one's side.

At this stage, if your internal battery is completely depleted, find a way to give yourself the space and time to do whatever you need to recharge it—sleep as long as your body wants to sleep, go to a friend's home to be taken care of, get a massage, spend time in prayer or meditation, write in a journal, visit a place in nature or a museum that you love, or do something else to balance your energy. Many studies have shown that extreme exhaustion can have the same effect as inebriation; if you do not take steps to replenish and rebalance, you risk possibly having an accident or injury.

Sadness, Anger, Aloneness, and Other Strong Emotions

After the period of exhaustion or numbness, you may feel enormous waves of sadness come over you, more powerful than any sadness you have felt before. This is only logical, for you have probably experienced a greater loss than you have ever experienced before. In addition to thinking about your loved one and missing him or her, you may also relive the experience of loss of other relatives, friends, or beloved family pets. Grief has a way of dredging up from the bottom of your being layers of sadness that have been covered by the silt of daily life.

One friend commented that after having gone through such a whirlwind of activity in the final days of caregiving, and then the intensity of organizing and participating in the funeral and burial services, she was struck by a profound sense of silence and aloneness, almost like being in a desert.

If your loved one spent their final days in a hospital or nursing home that did not meet your expectations and standards, or if you experienced difficult interactions with family members, you may also experience anger or resentment and find yourself reliving past traumatic events or having recurring, troublesome dreams or insomnia. If this is so, counseling, meditation, or a grief support group can be helpful.

Feeling the Presence of Your Departed Loved One

I have spoken to many people who have had experiences of feeling as though their departed loved one was communicating with them. *One person felt as if her sister was communicating through the song of a bird that began to visit their back yard only after her sister died. Another friend told me that the night after her sister died, she experienced a physical sensation, quite pleasant, which indicated that her sister was making contact with her. She told me that her sister's son had a different experience, but he also felt that she was making contact. She believed that this happened because she and her nephew were not there at the moment of death and her sister was seeking them out to say good-bye and let them know that everything was OK!*

Another friend said that he had had several occasions in which a departed relative or friend's energy seemed to be present, and in which he heard a voice speaking to him, offering guidance that seemed to be very much in keeping with the departed person's wisdom and experience.

Yet another friend spoke of a time when she was away on a consulting job, a high pressured assignment in a far off city, taking place on the eve of her grandfather's death. She had told herself not to think of him, worrying that it would bring up too many emotions at a time she needed focus and strength. She managed to avoid thinking about her grandfather until she laid her head on the pillow of the hotel bed. Then, she heard her grandfather's voice telling her to get up and sit in a chair while he talked with her. She did so, and her grandfather's voice offered insight to her that put the next day's assignment into perfect order. She was able to go to sleep and rest deeply, fully prepared for the day's work ahead.

I hope that it will comfort you to hear that others have had such experiences and that they can be healing and affirming, especially if the loss has felt very deep.

Honoring Your Grieving Process

As the weeks go by, you will find yourself riding a roller coaster of highs and lows happening in rapid succession. A song on the radio, a whiff of spring air after a rain shower, the sound of children laughing, anything familiar and dear to you can trigger your sadness. So, too, will the holidays and holy days that come before you. The empty place at the table on your birthday, no one to remember the famous recipe for the glazed sweet potatoes at Thanksgiving, a space next to you as you sit in temple or church on a high holy day or at the next wedding, may all trigger sadness welling up within you with unexpected force. Some families find it helpful to establish new holiday or holy day traditions, such as going away to celebrate holidays or to someone else's home, and some need to feel the "empty space" and the feelings that come with it. There is no "right" or "wrong" way to grieve, so do whatever you feel is right for you.

It is also not uncommon for you to have dreams about giving care to your loved one, or to wake up with something in your mind that you know you need to buy before driving to the nursing home, only to remember that you don't need to go to the nursing home anymore. At this stage, you may wonder to yourself, "Who am I if I am not a caregiver?"

The temptation may come to you to make major changes in your life, such as a geographical move or taking a new job, in order to fill the void of no longer being a caregiver or to cover over the sadness and feelings that are emerging. Several trusted counselors have said that they recommend not making major changes within the first year of a death, for if the changes are used to cover over the pain of grief, the pain will probably only emerge at a later time. Also, major change, even positive change, is a stressor. Taking on the additional stress of moving house and home, or the sharp learning curve that goes with taking a new job, when you are physically and emotionally exhausted is probably not what your body and mind need. You may be better off to think about your future and take small steps to investigate a major move or job change in the months following the death, but postpone the actual change until you have experienced a longer time frame, perhaps a one-year cycle of holidays and holy days, birthdays, anniversary dates, and changing seasons, or perhaps a longer amount of time.

Writing in a journal, doing artwork, or creating in whatever other way appeals to you may be particularly helpful as a way of noting your changing feelings and thoughts, as well as setting down images or words that describe alternative visions for your future.

As you approach or pass the one-year anniversary of your loved one's death, you might feel as if a large weight is being lifted from your shoulders or you may experience a feeling of spaciousness in your life that you hadn't had before. It is then that new green shoots of possibility begin to make themselves known. It took a full year after the death of my mother before I experienced this spaciousness and felt the luxury of evening hours available for reading and writing, along with other forgotten pastimes.

Whatever your grieving looks like or feels like, I hope that you find a way to honor your rhythms and cycles and to record them, if you wish.

CHAPTER THIRTEEN

NOW WHAT? HOW TO USE YOUR KNOWLEDGE TO HELP OTHERS

- Become a Hospice Volunteer
- Join a Support Group, Online Community, or Blog
- Become a Social Change Activist
- Some "Big Picture" Ideas

Once your role as a caregiver is over and you have taken time to grieve and adjust to your life without your loved one, I encourage you to consider how you can help others who are caring for dying loved ones.

There are many ways to be helpful, some quite informal. For example, if you hear that a friend's parent or spouse is dying, you can offer to be a "listening ear" to the caregiver or to sit with their loved one. Having been through this process yourself, you will be much more helpful than someone who has not been a caregiver before.

Become a Hospice Volunteer

You may also want to explore becoming a hospice volunteer, to pass along the help that was given to you by volunteers during your loved one's illness. Most hospices offer training programs that provide information concerning hospice services and death and dying, to prepare those who wish to serve others as hospice volunteers. If you do not wish to be a hospice volunteer who visits with families, there are other ways in which to assist your hospice, such as helping with fundraising events, mailings, or other office tasks.

Join a Support Group, Online Community, or Blog

There are grief support groups and internet communities or blogs available, wherever you may live. If you are drawn to the idea of joining a group that meets either in-person or online, you can check with your local hospice or use a search engine to search for "grief support groups." Some grief groups have a religious approach, some are facilitated by counseling professionals, and others are peer-facilitated. As with searching for professional counseling help, be sure to inquire about the mission and purpose of the group, the qualifications of the facilitators, and any costs or commitments associated with joining the group. As with choosing a psychotherapist, you may want to investigate several groups before deciding upon one; even if you choose one, if it doesn't work out, you can try another one.

Another option is to consider forming a group through your workplace or religious denomination, or in your local community.

During the time in which I was caring for my mother, and after her death, I realized that a number of colleagues in my workplace were also grieving the loss of loved ones. We formed a "grief group" that met during our lunch hour every other week in a private room. In that confidential setting, attendees were safe to share their experiences with others who were grieving the loss of loved ones who had died, whether recently or many years in the past.

I am very grateful for the support of that group. Although it only met for a few months, it offered support to me at a time when I needed to know that others were also going through their journeys of grief. Hearing others' stories also affirmed that each of us has her own journey of grief, and that journey cannot be fit into any set schedule.

Become a Social Change Activist

Everyone with whom I have spoken during the writing of this book agrees with me about one thing—changes in the present health care delivery system are desperately needed in order to provide low cost, high quality care for all persons at the end of life.

If you are not satisfied with the end-of-life options that currently exist, and you want to have more options for your end-of-life care, now is the time to consider how you can help to shape the future of end-of-life care. The actions that you take to advocate to create more and better options for end-of-life care will benefit you and will benefit the generations to come.

There are many ways to become active: You may want to write an editorial, contact your legislator to draft or pass legislation, or file an incident or grievance report with the state board that oversees the type of facility at which your loved one lived. Each of these actions can give you a sense of working for the greater good.

The changes that I would like to see on a structural level are as follows:

- Funding of Medicare and Medicaid must increase. The current funding levels do not support respectful care of residents or respectful treatment of workers.

- Medicare and Medicaid funding for rehabilitative and post-rehabilitative care must be made available for home care and custodial care, rather than only certified nursing home care.

- Medicare regulations and discharge protocols that require families to provide 24 hour a day care after the patient's discharge from Medicare-paid rehabilitative care should be eliminated. Few families can afford the $13,000-$20,000 per month cost of 24 hour at home care. Many patients are told by discharge planners that they must enter nursing homes or risk the loss of Medicare benefits for a period of time.

- Funding through Medicare must be made available to families without the "three day hospital stay" requirement that elimi-nates many from receiving such coverage.

- Better coordination of services is needed on regional and local levels so that persons needing services can find them easily.

- More federal and state funding must be allocated to agencies that investigate reports of nursing home abuse and patient safety issues. Currently in Massachusetts, there are thousands of nursing home complaints that have yet to be investigated, and only a few investigative staff to do the investigations.

- Federal and state oversight is needed to protect families who report nursing home problems from being pressured by the nursing home administration to move their loved ones from the nursing home. *This pressure is very real. I have seen it happen in one of the "best" nursing homes in my area. Unfortunately, currently there is no process to address efforts to silence those who wish to improve the health and safety conditions of nursing homes.*

Some "Big Picture" Ideas

Personally, I believe that many more changes are needed, beyond these immediate structural and legislative changes, to create adequate systems and processes for offering adequate end of life care to all dying persons. I will list eight ideas here, in the hopes that readers will comment on the blog on my website: www.caringfordyinglovedones.com and help to develop the ideas that have merit or invent new ideas with more merit.

1) A "hospice bank system," where persons trained as hospice volunteers could "invest" substantial amounts of time, anywhere from 5-30 hours per week, being companions and sitters for hospice patients, and then "withdraw" volunteer hours when they need them for their own care, perhaps decades later. This could operate as an extension of the current hospice volunteer programs at local hospices. Perhaps the family being helped could contribute a minimal fee, such as $1-2 per hour, to the hospice for scheduling the volunteers and keeping records of the hours banked by the volunteers. If this was successful on a local level, perhaps a national organization of hospices could make it possible for senior volunteers to have portability of hours, should they end up moving from their original location to a new one.

2) A "buy back" real estate program, equivalent to the type of "paid-up" death benefit that insurances companies give persons with terminal illness who wish to cash in their insurance plans before they die. Currently, "reverse mortgages" charge large upfront origination fees of up to $15,000, plus mortgage insurance on the appraised value, as well as mortgage interest and additional monthly fees. This can make for a very costly transaction. Perhaps HUD or another federal agency could offer a less expensive option with low up-front costs, such as buying the person's house and allowing the person to stay at home and rent from the agency until the time of their death. This would make available the largest asset that most homeowners have in their lives, the paid-up equity in their own home.

3) Development of a new classification for workers who are "live-in hospice workers" (equivalent to "nannies") so that people could hire

live-in CNAs and the room and board would be factored into their compensation.

An elderly friend wanted to stay in her home. As she reached the age of 90, she began speaking more in her native tongue, Polish. The mixture of Polish and English was not problematic at first, then more challenging, as those of us who knew no Polish struggled to understand her. We struggled to find CNAs who could speak both English and Polish; most could speak only English, and one could speak only Polish. We wished we had been able to hire someone from Poland who wanted to come to the U.S. and be a live-in helper with a temporary visa status.

4) Expanded "home sharing" networks whereby elders with large homes or empty apartment rooms could offer rent free living to prescreened persons, in exchange for a limited amount of work such as light housekeeping, shopping or cooking. This is not a new idea. There are agencies that make such matches in some areas of the country, but there is a large need for this type of match-making in order to provide services to elders and provide low cost living expenses to graduate students and others in transition in their lives.

5) Increased dialogue about "quality of life" and "quantity of life." As the pharmaceutical and medical advancements have extended human life by decades during the last century, we have created a situation where millions of people are now living for years and even decades in a state that is "not really living, not yet dying," where there is little enjoyment or quality of life. I suggest that we begin by questioning the orientation of our system of medicine, pharmaceuticals, and health insurance, which is focused mostly on "fixing bodies that are broken" rather than educating and supporting people in developing and sustaining healthy eating, exercise, sleep, stress management, and other wellness habits. The old adage "an ounce of prevention is worth a pound of cure" is very wise, yet our current system pays more for medical care in the final two years of a person's life than in the 70 or 80 or 90 years beforehand. A much greater emphasis on providing adequate nutrition and health care for all pregnant mothers, infants, and young children, and educating children and adults of all ages as to the responsibility of caring for one's body and mind, is desperately needed.

6) More dialogue about the ways to eliminate inequalities in health and health care based on race and socio economic class. Our present health care system sustains huge disparities of health and health care between rich, white persons and poor people and persons of color. These differences are also permitted through policies that allow low income areas to used as dumping grounds for toxic materials and as sites for industries that pollute the air and water.

7) We ought to use television, movies, other media, and face-to-face settings to talk more about death and dying, so that people who have never been close to death can examine their fears and learn about dying from others who have been caregivers. We have gone from a culture where people died at home and were waked in the parlor, only 100 years ago, to a culture where death is shut away and feared to such an extent that most people are "death deniers."

8) We ought to continue to talk thoughtfully and civilly about the issue of choosing to end one's own life, realizing that this is an issue about which people have strident beliefs on both sides. Currently, only one state, the state of Oregon, permits physician-assisted suicide, yet in many polls, the majority of Americans express their support for individuals with terminal diagnoses to have the power to end their own lives in a painless way, without interference from those who wish to stop them and with adequate safeguards in place to prevent abuse of such freedom by medical staff or anyone else.

I hope that these ideas stimulate your own ideas concerning life, quality of life, and caring for loved ones. Please visit my website: www.caringfordyinglovedones.com to post your own ideas and to view others' posts, so that the dialogue can continue to take place on these important topics.

Resources

A wide range of support services is available to you as a caregiver that did not exist a decade or two ago. Your journey as a caregiver will be made easier to the extent that you avail yourself of these resources.

I encourage you to buy additional copies of *Caring for Dying Loved Ones: A Helpful Guide for Families and Friends* from Levellers Press, www.levellerspress.com, the worker-owned publishing house that decided to publish this book. Your support of Levellers Press will allow them to provide other authors with the chance to share their ideas with readers everywhere.

If you wish to buy other books listed here, I hope that you will buy them through your independent, locally-owned bookstore. If you no longer have an independently owned bookstore, I encourage you to make your purchases online from Food for Thought Books (www.foodforthoughtbooks.com.) Or, pick up the phone to call an organization that can offer the advice, support, or services that you need, or visit the website listed for more information. Additional resources, and updates of these resources, will be posted at www.caringfordyinglovedones.com.

Adult Day Care

A link to all available senior care services may be found on www.medicare.gov

A trusted adult day care facility in Western Massachusetts is: ThayerCare, Inc. 49 Middle St., Hadley, MA 01035 www.thayercare.com, 413-584-0300 bthayer@thayercare.com

AIDS— *Acquired Immune Deficiency Disease/HIV*

www.aids.gov is the official US government web site for AIDS. www.aidsinfo.nih.gov is the site on the National Institutes of Health

www.cdc.gov/hiv/resources/factsheets is the Centers for Disease Control information site on AIDS

Alzheimer's and Dementia

Alzheimer's Association, www.alz.org, 1-800-272-3900. Since there are so many similarities between persons with vascular dementia and Alzheimer's disease, I recommend that all persons helping loved ones with dementia go to www.alz.org for information.

Mace, Nancy L., M.A., and Peter V. Rabins, M.D., Ph.D. *The 36-Hour Day, a Family Guide to Caring for Persons with Alzheimer's Disease, Related Dementing Illness, and Memory Loss in Later Life.* New York, NY: Warner Books. 1991.

Avoiding Nursing Homes

Bennett, Clifford, Ph.D. *Senior Power, Your Last Chance to Avoid Languishing in a Nursing Home Bed.* Northampton, MA: Alward Publications. 2007. Available by direct order for $22, including shipping. Make check for payable to: Life Systems, c/o Tracey Bennett, 139 Mayfair Ave, Springfield, MA 01104. *Author note: I highly recommend this book to readers. Dr. Bennett, a nursing home administrator, signed himself into an out-of-state nursing home to experience firsthand what nursing home life was like. His story, documenting his profound depression and the stories of fellow residents, was the basis for his doctoral thesis and is a "must read" for anyone considering nursing home care for their loved ones.*

Cancer

American Cancer Society www.cancer.org, 1-800-227-2345.

Cancer Connection, Inc. www.cancer-connection.org, POB 60452, Florence, MA 01062. 413-586-1642. This Western Massachusetts nonprofit organization is a wonderful model of an organization that provides free workshops, support groups, and complementary healing modes (art, music, massage therapy, Reiki healing, acupuncture) to those with cancer and their families.

National Cancer Institute (NCI), www.cancer.gov, 1-800-422-6237.

Caregiver Rejuvenation

For those who can afford to take an "away vacation," I recommend the following site, which lists retreat centers of great beauty: www.powersofplace.com, (Even viewing the photographs is restful!)

Children

The Compassionate Friends, www.compassionatefriends.org, "To assist families toward the positive resolution of grief following the death of a child of any age" has 625 chapters, in the U.S. 877-969-0010.

Zucker, Robert. *The Journey Through Grief and Loss: Helping Yourself and Your Child When Grief Is Shared.* St. Martin's Press. 2009. Robert Zucker's personal website, www.robertzucker.com, has many articles concerning families, children, grief and loss.

Communicating with Relatives and Friends

CaringBridge, www.caringbridge.org, a nonprofit organization set up to provide free websites so that families dealing with the illness of a loved one can easily communicate with one another

Facebook, www.facebook.com (a free way to create a website)

Skype, www.skype.com, (video/phone conversation software. All that is needed is a computer, a small video camera ("webcam", costing $40 or less at Radio Shack or any other electronic equipment provider), and Skype software, to enjoy video-telephone conversations.

Twitter, www.twitter.com, (texting software to use with a phone, to relay short text messages or view messages from others)

Death and Dying

www.growthhouse.org, "free access to over 4,000 pages of high quality educational materials about end-of-life care, palliative medicine, and hospice care."

Kubler-Ross, Elisabeth, Dr. The late Dr. Kubler-Ross was the author of many books about death and dying. Search via her name on any internet search engine to find the complete list. Hearing her speak at a conference in 1983 about the concepts in her book *On Death and Dying* began my process of thinking about death and dying issues.

Kubler-Ross, Elisabeth. *On Death and Dying.* New York: Touchstone, Simon & Schuster.

Kubler-Ross, Elisabeth. *Death, The Final Stage of Growth.* New York: Touchstone, Simon & Schuster.

Levine, Stephen. *A Year to Live: How to Live This Year as if It Were Your Last.* New York: Bell Tower. 1997.

EMDR—*Eye Movement Desensitization and Reprocessing*

www.emdria.org (A counseling technique for healing trauma)

Funeral Planning

Funeral Consumers Alliance, www.funerals.org, is "a federation of nonprofit consumer education societies protecting a consumer's right to choose a meaningful, dignified, affordable funeral since 1963." Their information kit "Before I Go You Should Know" is a 16 page funeral planning guide in a bright blue plastic folder. They also have extensive information concerning funerals, burials, caskets, and cremation, as well as updates on their activist efforts to create more options for funeral service consumers.

International Order of the Golden Rule, www.ogr.org, An association of selected "… privately owned funeral homes that demonstrate their commitment to funeral service through dedication to their community's needs." Member funeral homes must be peer-reviewed and must abide by high ethical standards and "*a commitment to Service measured not by gold, but by the Golden Rule.*" The "Information for Families" link has a Golden Rule Funeral Home search function.

International Cemetery, Cremation and Funeral Association, www.iccfa.com, is primarily a professional association website, but the "Information for Consumers" section has some eye-opening information concerning what happens to money upon prepayment of expenses. It is also instructive to visit the "Café" side of the website to see what issues are of concern to cemetery operators, such as news of recent lawsuits.

National Funeral Directors Association website, www.nfda.org, has many articles and resources for funeral directors and the general public, as well as a funeral home search function.

National Funeral Directors and Morticians Association, Inc., www.nfdma.com, is the oldest organization that was started by and for African American funeral directors. Tel: 800-434-0958 to locate member funeral homes.

Sublette, Kathleen, and Flagg, Martin. *Final Celebrations: A Guide for Personal and Family Funeral Planning.* Ventura, California: Pathfinder Publishing. 1992.

Grief

Compassionate Friends, www.compassionatefriends.org, is a non-profit organization that exists "To assist families toward the positive resolution of grief following the death of a child of any age." 600 chapters, in the US and 30 countries.

Akner, Lois F., CSW with Catherine Whitney. *How to Survive the Loss of a Parent, A guide for Adults.* New York: Harper. 1993.

Callanan, Maggie and Kelley, Patricia. *Final Gifts: Understanding the Special Awareness, Needs, and Communication of the Dying.* New York, Bantam Books. 1997.

Colgrove, Melba. *How to Survive the Loss of a Love.* New York: Prelude Press, 1993.

Zucker, Robert. *The Journey Through Grief and Loss: Helping Yourself and Your Child When Grief Is Shared.* St. Martin's Press. 2009. Please also see his personal website, www.robertzucker.com, where he has several free articles available for viewing.

Health Care Proxy Form

www.betterending.org, has information in English, Spanish, and Vietnamese

Heart Disease

American Heart Association, www.heart.org, 1-800-242-8721.

HIPAA—*Health Insurance Portability and Accountability Act*

The U.S. Department of Health and Human Services is the website where you will find information about the HIPAA Privacy Rule, passed to protect the privacy of individually identifiable health care information, the HIPAA Security Rule, that sets national standards for the security of electronically protected health information, and the confidentiality provisions of the Patient Safety Rule, which protects identifiable information being used to analyze patient safety events and improve patient safety. The HIPAA authorization form is available at:
www.hhs.gov/ocr/privacy/hipaa/understanding/index.html.

Hospice

The sites below have many helpful articles on end-of-life topics such as pain, nutrition, and hydration as well as hospice locator links.

Hospice & Palliative Care Federation of Massachusetts
www.hospicefed.org, 781-255-7077.

Hospice Foundation of America
www.hospicefoundation.org, 800-854-3402.

National Hospice & Palliative Care Organization (NHPCO)
www.nhpco.org, 703-837-1500.

www.hospicedirectory.org, is an online directory of hospices.

Hospice of the Fisher Home, www.fisherhome.org, 413-549-2751. This live-in hospice in North Amherst, MA has cared for two of my friends. This home truly models "resident-centered care."

Home Health Care Agencies

(Use an internet search engine to look up "VNA" Or "Home Health Care Agencies" or "Hospice")

I highly recommend the following two agencies, which serve Western Massachusetts. (You may find it helpful to see their websites, even if you do not live locally).

Barton's Angels, www.bartonsangels.com, POB 343, Northampton, MA 01060 413-582-0220.

O'Connell Care at Home, www.opns.com, 14 Bobala Rd, Suite 1B, Holyoke, MA 01040 413-533-1030.

Living Will (Medical Directive)

See appendices A and B (pages 167-172) for sample language that you can consider including in a living will. Also, visit www.nolo.com as a website for investigating low cost and no cost legal resources and forms.

Medicare and Medicaid

www.medicare.gov, 1-800-633-4227 (TTY 877-486-2048), is the master site (and telephone number) at which you can find out everything about Medicare and Medicaid plans, including costs and benefits of different plans ("Medicare Options Compare" tool) . You will also find a list of alternatives to nursing home care, including Socially Managed Care Plans and PACE (both of these are only offered in specific regions), and links to agencies serving the elderly, including www.eldercare.gov, 1-800-486-2048. If you are considering skilled nursing home care, I encourage you to download the 68 page booklet about choosing a nursing home, read the criteria for skilled nursing home care under Medicare plans, and check the nursing home comparison database, "Compare Nursing Homes in Your Area" (with a five star rating system).

Multiple Sclerosis

www.nationalmssociety.org, 1-800-344-4867

Music Thanatology

See, www.mtai.org/index.php?whatis, for an explanation of how persons trained in music thanatology use harp and voice to "lovingly serve the physical, emotional, and spiritual needs of the dying…" Also, see www.caringfordyinglovedones.com

Near Death Experiences

Atwater, P. M. 0H. *The Big Book of Near-Death Experiences: The Ultimate Guide to What Happens When We Die.* Charlottesville, VA: Hampton Roads Publishers. 2007.

Moody, Raymond, Jr. *Life After Life.* New York: Bantam. 1975.

Nursing Homes

www.medicare.gov/nhcompare is the governmental site that contains a number of excellent resources about evaluating and choosing a nursing home, as well as a database of ratings for nursing homes.

Pain Management

The American Cancer Association, www.cancer.org.

Hospice Foundation of America, www.hospicefoundation.org.

Obituaries Online

On the two sites below, you can sign online guest books or search for past obituaries. Results for searches prior to 1995 can be spotty.

www.legacy.com

www.tributes.com

Parkinson Disease

National Parkinson Foundation www.parkinson.org, 1-800-327-4545.

Physiological Aspects of Dying

www.growthhouse.org provide educational materials about end-of-life care, palliative medicine, and hospice care, including descriptions of the end stages of specific diseases.

Nuland, Sherwin D. *How We Die.* New York: Vintage Books, a Division of Random House, Inc.1995. Written by a physician, this book gives a detailed explanation of what happens on a bodily level as someone dies due to cancer, AIDS, Alzheimer's disease, heart disease, and strokes.

Psychological and Spiritual Aspects of Dying

Dalia Lama, His Holiness the. Translated and Edited by Jeffrey Hopkins, PhD. *Advice on Dying and Living a Better Life.* New York: Atria Books. 2002.

Kubler-Ross, Elisabeth. *On Death and Dying.* New York: Touchstone, Simon & Schuster. (1997)

Kubler-Ross, Elisabeth. *Death, The Final Stage of Growth.* New York: Touchstone, Simon & Schuster. (1986)

Levine, Stephen. *A Year to Live, How to Live This Year As If It Were Your Last.* New York: Bell Tower, Member of the Crown Publishing Group. 1997.

Tobin, Daniel R., MD, with Karen Lindsey. *Peaceful Dying, the Step-by-Step Guide to Preserving Your Dignity, Your Choice, and Your Inner Peace at the End of Life.* Cambridge, MA: Da Capo Press, a member of the Perseus Books Group. 1999

Stroke

National Stroke Association, www.stroke.org, 1-800-787-6537

Staying at Home

Use a search engine or look up in your local phone directory under "VNA" or "Visiting Nurse Association" or "Hospice," or your local hospital, which might have the hospice or VNA listed as a department within it. Also, look up under your city or town name, for example, "Chicopee Visiting Nurses."

"Village to Village" self-help membership organizations, www.vtvnetwork.org, The first nonprofit neighborhood "village" organization started in 2001 in Beacon Hill in Boston, (www.beaconhillvillage.org).These mutual-aid societies, funded with membership dues, offer services to persons 50 or older who wish to stay in their homes but are no longer self-sufficient. Call 617-299-9NET for more information.

Women's Health

Dr. Christiane Northrup. www.drnorthrup.com is a site containing articles and resource books focusing on women's health. Her latest books are on various topics related to menopause. Fax: (207) 846-8953

Veterans Benefits

For complete information regarding veterans death benefits, call your local veterans office, or go to the website, www.va.gov, or call 1-800-827-1000.

Veteran grave marker. To find out more information about grave markers for veterans, call 1-800-697-6947 from 8 am until 5 pm, Monday through Friday, except federal holidays, or consult the website, www.cem.va.gov.

APPENDIX A

Sample Language for a Living Will

The following language is a general statement of wishes for end of life care that can be written into a living will:

If at any time my attending physician should determine that I have a terminal condition where the application of life-prolonging procedures would serve only to artificially prolong the dying process, I direct that such procedures be withheld or withdrawn, and that I be permitted to die naturally with only the administration of medication or the performance of any medical procedure deemed necessary to provide me with comfort care or to alleviate pain.

Specific wishes:

I specifically direct that the following instructions be followed, if my physician determines that a cure is not possible, there is no expectation of recovery to a state of wellness, and the course of my illness is such that prolonged suffering and incapacitation are likely and expected before death (please write your initials in front of all that you wish to have apply to you and your care):

___ Treatment should be given to keep me comfortable and relieve pain, even if this treatment might dull my consciousness and indirectly shorten my life.

___ If my heart stops, I do not want it to be restarted through chest compressions, drugs, electric shocks or by any other means used to revive a person who is at the point of dying.

___ If I stop breathing, I do not want to have a breathing tube inserted into my throat and be connected to a respirator (mechanical breathing).

___ I do not want to be placed on kidney dialysis (cleaning the blood through a machine or by fluid passing through my belly) if dialysis will simply prolong my life on a temporary basis.

___ I do not wish to receive blood transfusions or blood products if these will only prolong my life on a temporary basis.

___ I do not wish to receive invasive diagnostic procedures or surgical procedures if these are expected to only prolong my life temporarily; or, if there is little likelihood of my condition and quality of life substantially improving as a result of these procedures; or, if the discomfort, complications, and risks associated with such procedures outweigh the possible benefits.

___ My doctor may withhold or stop treatment or medication that only serves to extend the dying process. Treatment or processes that may be withheld can include, but not be limited to:

___ If I am not able to drink, I do not want to receive fluids through intravenous solutions (a needle placed into a vein).

___ If I am not able to feed myself or swallow food, I do not wish to allow a tube to be inserted into my mouth or my nose, or surgically inserted elsewhere into my body, to give me liquids or food.

___ If I have a fever or infection, I do not want antibiotics or other medications administered to me by any manner simply to prolong my life, unless these medications are necessary in order to alleviate my pain and make me more comfortable.

___ I would like to die at home with hospice care or in a hospice residence, if at all possible.

___ If I am in a nursing home, hospital, or any setting other than at home, I would like to die under the care of hospice.

___ Unless necessary for my comfort, I would prefer NOT to be hospitalized.

___ Unless necessary for my comfort, I would prefer NOT to be admitted to a nursing home or other institutional care facility, unless it is a hospice residence

___ If possible, I wish to be an organ/tissue donor

___ Any organs or tissues that can be of help to others.

___ Donations of only the following organs or tissues

___ I do NOT wish to have the following organs or tissues donated:

____ I wish to have my body, or any part of my body that can be useful to scientific or medical research, be donated for such purposes, provided that this request be made in writing and authorized by my medical health care agent in writing, and that there be no cost to my family or estate for doing so.

____ I do not wish to have any parts of my body or any tissues taken for scientific or medical research or other purposes, unless my medical health care agent has expressly been asked in writing and has granted permission in writing.

____ I do not wish to have an autopsy performed after my death, unless required by law to do so.

Please have the person sign below in the presence of two witness, who are not the health care agent of alternative agent.

Signed: _____ Date: _____

Print Name: _____

Witness signature _____

Witness name (print) _____

Witness signature _____

Witness name (print) _____

APPENDIX B

Additional Sample Language for a Living Will

The following language is included in my own living will. I include it here, because I have given care to loved ones who were not in "vegetative states," but who were nevertheless extremely incapacitated through stroke, end-stage heart or lung disease, cancer, or other degenerative diseases or terminal illnesses.

This has made me realize that I wanted to craft my Living Will to be far more explicit and specific concerning my end of life medical directive, beyond addressing "vegetative state" conditions.

Please feel free to use or modify the wording below, to meet your needs.

Please place your initials before whichever statements below you wish to include in your Living Will as statements of your own wishes:

___ It is very important to me that I am able to communicate verbally with those I love, and that I am able to at least partially care for myself. If I am not alert, active and of sound mind, I would not want to be kept alive, including by feeding tubes or IV fluids, except as to tide me over during a period of acute illness or following an accident or surgery, but only if recovery were likely.

___ I do not feel that life should be prolonged at all costs. I recognize that we all have to die of something, and I hope to die with dignity, and with my pain controlled, when the time comes. I ask my health care agents to make my decisions in light of this.

___ In the case of a stroke or other serious and chronic condition where I may not be in a vegetative state but cannot express my wishes, I hope never to be put into a nursing home where my freedom to eat, sleep, move, be alone, go the bathroom, or express my emotions will be in any way restricted via mechanical, medicinal, or procedural means.

___ I would rather stop eating and drinking and curtail my own life, than to be subjected to others' power over me in terms of eating, sleeping, being where I want to live, and in whatever condition I want to be in. If I am not able to voice my wants and wishes, and I purse my lips, close my mouth, or turn my head away from food that is offered to me, that is an expression of the fact that I no longer want to eat or drink, and this wish on my part should be honored. At this point, I wish comfort care only and wish you to commence pain relieving medications.

____ It is specifically repugnant to me to have the prospect of someone forcing me to sit or lie down while tethered (or on an alarmed pad), either in bed or in a wheelchair or other chair, so that I cannot stand up, or be made to sit or lie in bed in hallways and common areas of a nursing home or hospital, so that I could be watched by staff, rather than being able to be in a private space, enjoying quiet and/or solitude.

____ It is unacceptable to me that I might ever be forced to conform to a sleeping schedule or a toilet schedule (or to be put into diapers and left to sit in my own urine or excrement) to accommodate the convenience of staff.

____ If I am not able to make my own decisions, to feed and to care for myself, or to dictate who will care for me and how, to enjoy life, to interact with others as I wish, and to be of useful service in the world, then I willingly want to go on the great mystery beyond this life, knowable only through the gateway of death.

____ I do not wish to be utterly dependent on others, without being able to engage in activities and communicate in a way that is robust and meaningful to me. If I am not able to communicate my wishes, whether by writing, verbally, by nodding or shaking my head, by blinking my eyes, by pointing to words or images, by using a computer, or by any other means, then I would wish deliverance from this state of "non-living" by admittance to hospice care and administration of pain medication to ensure that I am pain-free, even if this hastens my death.

To Make your Living Will Legal

It is wise to consult the website of your state to educate yourself about the requirements for creating a living will. Massachusetts requires two witnesses who are not the healthcare agent or alternate agent. It is also recommended that the health care agent and alternate sign a form accepting the responsibility of being health care agent or alternate, although this is not required.

Afterword —
Why I Wrote This Book

My own path in helping relatives and friends in their final months, with all of its ups and downs, was the source of material for this book. I was 34 years old when I began to realize that my ailing 94-year old grandfather was dying. I was terrified of the prospect of being with him when he died, so I began asking my friends if they had ever been with someone as they had died. I spoke with more than 50 friends, relatives, and colleagues, some my age and some decades older than I, but none of the people with whom I spoke—including a doctor—had been present at the time of a person's death.

There was no hospice service available locally in 1986 that would enable my family to care for my grandfather at home once he became bed-ridden. It was a heart-breaking experience to travel with my grandfather in an ambulance as it carried him to a nursing home, as he struggled against restraints and yelled that he didn't want to leave his home. My explanation that it would be better for him to be in a nursing home did nothing to soothe his anger or his fear.

My grandfather lost the opportunity to live out his last days in the way he would have wanted to, and I lost the chance to be with him when he died. I swore then that I would not let the same thing happen to my grandmother when it came her time to leave this world.

In 1989, I had the chance to live out my convictions. I moved back to Western Massachusetts in order to be close to my 95-year old grandmother. Two years later, I became her hospice care coordinator and one of her primary caregivers. Taking care of her every evening after work and many hours on the weekends, and staying up all night one night a week to respond to her needs while working a full-time, demanding job as head of a nonprofit agency, was the most challenging experience of my life. It also proved to be the most meaningful and important experience of my life. In caring for my grandmother, I learned how important it was for her to die in her own home of 40 years, in her own bed, with her lilacs, irises, and her beautiful magnolia tree outside her window, and her beloved furniture, pictures, and personal belongings surrounding her.

Being with my grandmother as she experienced her final weeks, days, hours, and minutes showed me the changing nature of living and dying, with its unexpected turns and crises, memorable moments, and laughter. She was able to die the way she had lived, in peace and quiet, following her own rhythms and cycles of sleeping and waking, eating and not eating. Being with her at her moment of death was a deeply spiritual experience that completely removed my own fear of dying and prepared me for what was to come in caring for my parents and close friends in the years to come.

In 1999, my partner and I purchased a home four houses away from my elderly parents, in order to offer ongoing support to my ailing 85-year old father. What began as weekly visits became daily visits as my father ceased being able to be the "chief cook and bottle washer." In 2001, I had the opportunity to be my father's caregiver in his final weeks, days, and hours, and to be with him when he died. This time, no longer afraid of the moment of death, and having learned from a friend about death rituals in Lithuania (see page 142), I was able to be emotionally present with him both before and after his passing in a way that I would not have been able to imagine ten years earlier.

After caring for my father, I provided hospice care to two dear women friends. One friend was in her late 80s who suffered a massive stroke and lived her final two months in a rehabilitation hospital and a nursing facility. The other woman was my earliest childhood friend, who died in her own home at the age of 54 of pancreatic cancer. I was one of a loyal band of high school classmates and other close women friends who cared for her, with the support of hospice, and who designed and led her memorial service at her home.

Following my father's death in 2001, I provided care to my elderly mother in her home, at first on an infrequent basis and then on a daily and several times-daily basis. She suffered a stroke in July of 2005, and in September she moved to an assisted living unit. Only six weeks later, another stroke took its toll and she was moved to the skilled nursing unit, where she lived for more than a year. She spent the final three months of her life in a dementia unit. I continued to be her daily visitor and caregiver throughout the final chapter of her life. My mother died at the age of 91 with me by her side.

Each of these experiences in offering support to dying parents and friends has deepened my understanding of the blessings and burdens of being a caregiver and the importance of considering issues that will impact a dying person's ability to live out the final years, months, days, and hours of his life with dignity, respect, joy, and peace.

In the months following my mother's death, I found myself writing down insights and ideas related to my recent experiences in taking care of her, as well as rereading writing that I had done in caring for my grandparents, my father, and my friends. What began as journaling that I needed to do to process the intense experiences of being a caregiver, began to take the form of essays on topics, which then began to look like chapters that might make up a book. As I discussed my evolving project with close friends, they unanimously expressed support for me to think of writing and publishing a book that could be helpful to them and to others. The book that you hold in your hand is the result of their encouragement and my desire to support others on their caregiving journeys.

ACKNOWLEDGMENTS

*I wish to acknowledge the people who
most supported me as a caregiver.*

I am deeply grateful to my spouse and life partner, Jo Lower, who has unconditionally supported my caregiving of dying friends and relatives during our 18 years together. She visited my parents countless times and did hundreds of loads of laundry for them, provided solace in my grief, took care of our animals and our household in my absence, and urged me on in my advocacy of my mother and other nursing home residents.

I am also grateful to Sandy Zieminski, RN, for her exemplary care of her own mother and her unwavering support; Ralph and Linda Faulkingham, Michelle Landry, Mary Porcino, and the other members of our caregivers' support group for their invaluable advice and encouragement; other members of my family, biological and chosen, for their assistance; and members of "the grief group" at my workplace, for providing peer support as I shared my journey through grief.

I am grateful to have been a member of a small group of courageous and dedicated friends, including Nancy Carvalho, Cathy Rigali, L.P.N., and Cindy Strycharz as we cared for our friend in her final months of life and designed and led her memorial service.

I thank Irena Cade, who, by sharing with me her stories of caring for her dying mother in Lithuania, allowed me to envision that I would, one day, be prepared to lovingly wash my parents' and friends' bodies after their deaths.

I am grateful to Holly Hanson, who was instrumental in designing my mother's memorial service and who hosted the service and reception at her home, and to members of the Bahá'í community of South Hadley, Massachusetts, for being such good friends to my mother for more than 30 years.

I also wish to thank Melissa Tefft, LICSW, a gifted psychotherapist in Northampton, Massachusetts, whose EMDR therapy allowed me to heal traumatic incidents of my past. Through this therapy, I was able to become clear about my own goals as a caregiver, summon the strength and courage to speak my truth, and write and give the eulogies for my father, my mother, and three close friends at their respective memorial services.

I also wish to thank my writing coach, Mary Beth Averill, PhD, from Eugene, Oregon, www.writeonmba.com, for her superb advice and editing skill, and the following people who read drafts of this book and shared their comments: Magda Bechar, PhD, RN, Judith Ellenburg; Barbara Foster, MEd, Jo Goldman, MSW, LICSW; Georganne Greene; Attorney Bill Hart; Gail Hilyard; Jane Lekus; The Reverend Gloria G. Lomax, M.Ed. of the Hope Community Church in Amherst, Massachusetts; Edward Mazur; Carol McCarthy; Nora Wilcox, MD; Sandy Zieminski, RN, and Amy Zuckerman. I also thank others, who wished to remain anonymous, for sharing their stories of caregiving with me and allowing them to be used in this book.

Finally, I will always be grateful to my grandmother, my father, my mother, and the close friends who have allowed me to do the most sacred work of my life, caring for them in their most vulnerable moments and being with them in their final hours. Being their caregiver removed all fear of death for me, which is the greatest gift they could have given to me.

JOANNA LILLIAN BROWN *has been a caregiver to relatives and friends for nineteen years in addition to working full time in the fields of alumni relations and development. She lives in South Hadley, Massachusetts with her spouse, Jo Lower, their two dogs, Fenway and RBI, and their cat, Brindle.*